# A VEGAN ETHIC

Concise, accessible, and informative, *A Vegan Ethic* reminds us that compassion is not divisible, and neither should our activism be. Mark Hawthorne's empowering book explores why and how we can achieve social justice goals by working together and treating ourselves and others with compassion and respect. (And don't miss the helpful question-and-answer section!)
**Carol J. Adams**, author of *The Sexual Politics of Meat*

Now, more than ever, we need a smart and compassionate guide to connect animal activists with others working for social justice. *A Vegan Ethic* is that guide. It powerfully shows why we will be stronger when we work together for a better world for all. I hope every animal activist reads this book!
**Lori Gruen**, author of *Entangled Empathy: An Alternative Ethic for Our Relationships with Other Animals*

A consistently compassionate ethic can go far beyond not eating meat, eggs, and dairy. In *A Vegan Ethic*, Mark Hawthorne discusses how this ethic can connect with a much broader range of issues and shape a truly transformational view of the world.
**Jasmin Singer**, author of *Always Too Much and Never Enough* and co-host of *Our Hen House*

With *A Vegan Ethic*, Mark Hawthorne has created both a concise introduction to veganism and animal rights and an important call for vegans and animal advocates to be inclusive in their compassion. Drawing on the work of intersectional activists, Hawthorne demonstrates how spheres of oppression involving humans and nonhumans are connected and how we can all become agents of change. This is an important book that will

have a lasting impact on social justice.
**Kim Stallwood**, European director of the Animals & Society Institute and author of *Growl: Life Lessons, Hard Truths, and Bold Strategies from an Animal Advocate*

An animal advocate of 25 years, I continue to learn from Mark's work. His newest book is yet another testament to his skills and passion as a writer and as an effective voice for the oppressed. With his characteristic compassion, common sense, and practical guidance, Mark inspires reflection and conviction in his readers, moving them to change the way they think about and treat human and nonhuman animals.
**Colleen Patrick-Goudreau**, bestselling author of *The 30-Day Vegan Challenge* and *Vegan's Daily Companion*

Mark Hawthorne illuminates a path away from the oppression of animals, humans, and the environment, and toward a more just and peaceful society. *A Vegan Ethic* is food for the soul!
**Joyce Tischler**, founder of the Animal Legal Defense Fund

Mark Hawthorne provides a practical and accessible guide for veganism as an ethical framework. This book is an informative and helpful primer that demonstrates veganism is not about giving things up, but instead about opening ourselves up to the possibilities of a just and kinder world.
**Sangamithra Iyer**, author of *The Lines We Draw*

*A Vegan Ethic* is the most ambitious effort I've seen to put animal agriculture into its proper context as it relates to other systems of oppression. By understanding this context, activists will be better equipped to make crucial contributions when it comes to working to dismantle animal agribusiness.
**Erik Marcus**, publisher of Vegan.com

# A Vegan Ethic

Embracing A Life of Compassion Toward All

# A Vegan Ethic

Embracing A Life of Compassion Toward All

Mark Hawthorne

CHANGE
MAKERS
BOOKS

Winchester, UK
Washington, USA

First published by Changemakers Books, 2016
Changemakers Books is an imprint of John Hunt Publishing Ltd., Laurel House, Station Approach,
Alresford, Hants, SO24 9JH, UK
office1@jhpbooks.net
www.johnhuntpublishing.com
www.changemakers-books.com

For distributor details and how to order please visit the 'Ordering' section on our website.

Text copyright: Mark Hawthorne 2016

ISBN: 978 1 78535 402 1
Library of Congress Control Number: 2016931749

A CIP catalogue record for this book is available from the British Library.

Design: Stuart Davies

Printed in the USA by Edwards Brothers Malloy

We operate a distinctive and ethical publishing philosophy in all
areas of our business, from our global network of authors to
production and worldwide distribution.

# CONTENTS

## Also by Mark Hawthorne

Bleating Hearts: The Hidden World of Animal Suffering
Striking at the Roots: A Practical Guide to Animal Activism

# Acknowledgements

Every book, large or small, is a joint effort, and I owe much gratitude to those who have assisted me by reading early drafts and/or offering input or their support. My profound thanks to Carol J. Adams, Mollie Barker, Tara Baxter, Aurelia d'Andrea, Karen Emmerman, Lori Gruen, pattrice jones, Erik Marcus, Heidi Margocsy, Martin Rowe, Tom Ryan, and Kim Stallwood. I am also grateful to my friend and publisher, Tim Ward, for his guidance and for understanding the importance of a vegan ethic.

My views on the linked oppressions of species, gender, race, ecology, and sexuality have been informed by the work of many others, including Carol J. Adams, A. Breeze Harper, Marti Kheel, Greta Gaard, Lori Gruen, pattrice jones, Brian Luke, Norm Phelps, and most notably my wife, lauren Ornelas, who every day leads by example. Thank you, lauren, for sharing this life with me and helping me become a better person.

# Introduction

It doesn't seem so long ago that veganism was considered a fringe movement, regarded by many as an "extreme" way of eating and living practiced by those with an uncommon taste for tofu and brown rice. But as more and more people identify as vegan and avoid meat, eggs, dairy, and honey, they are becoming a driving economic force, and even major restaurant chains are doing their best to accommodate them by offering menus filled with plant-based fare. The general public is beginning to understand what a vegan means when she says she doesn't want to consume animals who were once living with their own dreams of happiness and freedom.

The beauty of veganism is that it's an antidote for so many of life's problems. In a world plagued by suffering, disease, and violence, a vegan lifestyle rejects the status quo and embraces compassion, nourishing us body and soul with healthy foods and a consideration for lives beyond our own. With *A Vegan Ethic*, we'll explore not only veganism, but animal rights, human rights, and the environment and then examine how we can nurture our better selves as we strive for social justice.

My own journey toward social justice began decades ago in Ladakh, amid the Himalayas of India. It was there, while living with a Buddhist family who grew their own food, that I learned what it meant to be a vegetarian. And it was there that I learned about the Chinese government's invasion of Tibet in 1950 and how, following a failed uprising in their homeland nearly a decade later, the Dalai Lama and thousands of his fellow Tibetans made the arduous trek over the mountains into India. This was the beginning of a protracted exodus from Tibet, and the population of Tibetan exiles around the world today is estimated to number about 150,000. I was deeply moved by the stories Tibetans told me, and I was welcomed into a refugee camp to better understand their plight. For several years after returning to the United States, I volunteered for a Tibet-support group, researching and writing articles for their newsletter.

All the while, I was examining my eating habits. After my time in Ladakh, I had stopped eating cows, chickens, and pigs, but I continued to consume fishes, milk from cows, and eggs from hens. I was living in denial, believing the lie that these "other" animals either had no feelings or "gave" their secretions for human use. But the more I learned about animal agriculture, the less I wanted to be among those who supported it. Confronting my habits meant recognizing that all animals want and deserve to live, and when we know this truth, I believe we have an obligation to do what we can to reduce suffering. And so I became an ethical vegan, reading widely, attending talks, and thinking critically about what it means to live compassionately.

One thing I took to heart is that part of living compassionately means not limiting one's empathy to a single group. If veganism is about doing your best to not harm *any* sentient life, we must logically extend that circle of compassion to human animals as well. One of the unfortunate aspects of the vegan/animal rights movement, however, is that in our struggle to liberate animals from farms, research, and captivity, we seldom see the connection between the exploitation of animals and the oppression of humans. Even those people who do see the link and are sympathetic with other social justice issues often believe they must ration their compassion and focus solely on animal causes. Worse are those who ignore the struggles of humanity because they feel disgusted with their own species and how we treat nonhumans. Anger and frustration are especially evident in online forums and on social media, where some "animal lovers" declare their hatred of humanity.

This is a deeply troubling barrier, though I understand the bitterness. Humans are responsible for committing countless atrocities against animals. But in frustration, many activists place animals above humans, rather than on the same plane, to the point that they have become misanthropes. It's easier for them to put all of their advocacy time and energy into helping a non-dominant group that can't advocate for themselves than to widen their circles of compassion and include oppressed people because humans, to their minds, are the problem and can speak for themselves. I cannot dissipate people's anger, but perhaps I can show them how that anger has been misdirected—that there is no freedom unless we all work together.

While the animal rights movement might be regarded as separate from other social justice movements, it, like the others, is part of the same fundamental struggle against domination, inequity, and exploitation. Only through cooperation and alliances among *all* liberation movements will we achieve our universal goal of emancipation.

In 1989, legal scholar Kimberlé Crenshaw introduced the term "intersectionality" to express the applicability of Black feminism to anti-discrimination law and thus explain how different forms or systems of oppression interact; it's a way of thinking about identity and its relationship to power, she said. This was at about the same time that author Carol J. Adams was using the term "interconnected oppressions" to describe how sexism, racism, and speciesism are linked. Indeed, with the publication of her groundbreaking 1990 book *The Sexual Politics of Meat*, Carol helped build a modern bridge between animal liberation and other movements.

Individuals and nonprofits have gradually been taking an interdisciplinary approach to social justice problems by discussing how animal rights issues intersect with human rights and how all movements might benefit. It's a premise that social justice activists, including those within the animal rights community, have actually acknowledged for decades. It's common for animal liberationists, for example, to say that speciesism—a prejudice that assigns greater moral significance to human animals than to other species—is like racism, sexism, and other forms of discrimination, which logically implies that all those things are morally unacceptable. Perhaps the most obvious illustration of this is animal rights as a feminist issue; both women's bodies and nonhuman animals' bodies are objectified as "things"—a "piece of meat" to be consumed. In particular, animal agriculture manipulates and exploits the bodies of female animals for eggs, milk, and breeding babies for meat.

Not surprisingly, women were early pioneers for social reform and animal liberation. In Victorian and Edwardian England, it was common for suffragists to be ethical vegetarians, and they championed the anti-vivisection cause. In fact, nineteenth-century animal activists in general seemed more apt to grasp the commonalities of oppression. Henry Bergh and Elbridge Thomas Gerry, for instance, founded both the American Society for the Prevention of Cruelty to Animals (1866) and the New York Society for the Prevention of Cruelty to Children (1874), the world's first organization for child protection.

Unfortunately, rather than becoming stronger, the alliances between animal advocates and social justice activists lost ground over the ensuing decades. The animal protection community too often focused on a single campaign, such as the treatment of working animals or assisting homeless dogs and cats, while other movements distanced themselves from the nonhuman crusade. This is changing, however slowly. More and more activists are recognizing the power of solidarity. Yet there is much resistance to this in the animal rights movement, with racism, sexism, classism, and other discriminatory, toxic attitudes poisoning our progress.

We gain nothing if we continue to ignore the universal spheres of oppression in orbit around us all—humans, nonhumans, everyone. We all lose. Doing our best not to cause harm or contribute to suffering is the central tenet of veganism, and as I argue in the following pages, fully embracing a life of compassion toward all is our best chance for creating the kind of world we dream of.

I want to be very clear that this book is a reflection of what I've learned from many activists and leaders in the animal rights and social justice communities, and I will refer to them and their work frequently, in both the text and the endnotes.

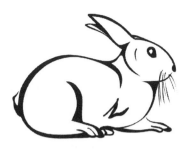

# Chapter 1

# On Animal Rights

*The way to right wrongs is to turn the light of truth upon them.*
—Ida B. Wells-Barnett

As I sat high in the stands of Pamplona's bullring and recovered from my run with the bulls, I felt a troubling call of my conscience. It was more of a whisper, really, but it was unwelcome and at first I ignored it. Below me, several young bulls were running loose in the arena, which was filled with scores of revelers like me who had just participated in the city's famed sprint through cobblestone streets. The hooligans were now engaged in what is known in Spain as a *vaquilla*—a spectacle that traditionally follows the bull run and apparently calls for the fiesta-goers to taunt smaller bulls and smack them with rolled-up newspapers.

Suddenly a nimble young bull scooped up a runner with his horns and tossed him over his back. That's when my conscience whispered to me again. It dawned on me that these animals—and the bulls I'd run with, who would die later that day in the bullring—deserve mercy, not misery. It was July of 1992, and up to that time, I'd never given much thought to the dignity or needs of animals. But that whisper was the voice of integrity tugging at my sleeve, and I couldn't shake it. A few months later, after an enlightening face-to-face encounter with a cow in India, I put the meat-eating phase of my life behind me and went vegetarian. It took another decade for me to go vegan, but when I did, the plight of animals became part of my world in a way that I never would have imagined possible. Now I'm the one tugging on sleeves.

Today, as an activist and ethical vegan, I look back on my experience in Pamplona with a combination of shame and gratitude. I am certainly not proud to have supported the blood "sport" of bullfighting. But being so close to bulls one moment and then confronting the horror of their fate the next helped me understand that we have an obligation to look out for the vulnerable, regardless of their species. It awakened something in me. Many of us have experiences like this. For some, it takes only one such moment to recognize our collective responsibility. For most of us, though, it's a more gradual process through which we decide what role compassion will play in our lives.

## Our Moral Contradictions

The essential quandary of the animal rights movement might be summed up in this question: Why do humans love some animals and eat (or otherwise abuse) others? According to the Humane Society of the United States, 47 percent of all households in the country have at least one dog and 46 percent have at least one cat—and other homes have many more—resulting in a population of some 83 million dogs and 95 million cats living with humans. Other countries, notably Australia, Canada, and England, have a similar affection for these animals. In Japan, many people prefer pets to parenthood, with dogs and cats far outnumbering children younger than 15. On top of this worldwide affinity for felines and canines are millions more rabbits, hamsters, rats, mice, birds, horses, and other pets. Most of these animals are treated like members of the family, often receiving birthday and holiday presents. They are carried about like infants. Some have social media accounts. They are outfitted in designer fashions and included in family portraits. We spend about US$60 billion a year feeding them and keeping them healthy, and we mourn their deaths—frequently with the same profound grief we experience over the loss of our dearest human loved ones. The status of pets has increased so much in our society that many animal lovers have taken to referring to them as *companion animals.*

On the other end of the spectrum are animals our culture eats. Needless to say, these chickens, fishes, pigs, cows, sheep, goats, turkeys, ducks, and geese are treated quite differently than the dogs and cats. Yet, imagine if our beloved companion animals were abused like animals in a farm: crammed into windowless sheds, lying in their own excrement, denied many of their natural instincts, their bodies mutilated, fed a toxic concoction of feed and pharmaceuticals to keep them alive, and then, finally, hauled for many miles to a slaughterhouse, where they witness the terrifying deaths of their fellows before they themselves are killed. These animals receive no love, let alone a special treat on their birthdays. Indeed, most of them are still babies when they are slaughtered.

Our relationship with other species is inconsistent, to say the least. But if our moral contradictions are troubling, relatively few people let on. Instead, they sleep under the dome of cognitive dissonance—a fancy term for the subtle discomfort we experience (often just a whisper) when holding two incompatible thoughts, or cognitions, at the same time. For example, millions of people smoke tobacco, despite knowing that smoking is bad for them. In the case of animals, people can alleviate cognitive dissonance by according animals moral status and going vegan, but only a small percentage of people have taken that course (so far).

The answer to our question, I think, as to why we as a society are able to love some animals and eat others, is that most people don't usually think of meat as coming from an animal—at least, they don't consciously process it that way. To them, meat is something you buy in the grocery store, sterile and removed from the violence of the animal's death, or order at a restaurant. I doubt they could live with themselves if they put pigs on the same level as dogs; in fact, that's why many omnivores (those who eat animal- and plant-based foods, which is to say most people) are so resistant to the animal rights message: it threatens to either remove animals from their diet (an old habit) or make them feel guilty for eating them.

Animal-consumers continue their habits with a clear conscience by rejecting the notion that animals are anything but mindless, emotionless creatures. It's difficult to eat someone when you accept that she or he has a personality, experiences pain, and wants to live. It makes it even harder to maintain moral ambivalence when you learn these same animals are good mothers who grieve the loss of their babies or that they become terrified when they see other animals being killed—it's not at all uncommon for frightened cows and pigs to escape a slaughter-house and literally run for their lives, though sadly very few end up in the safety of a sanctuary. Animal sentience is the most inconvenient truth of all.

Our cognitive dissonance extends beyond farmed animals to include those used for testing, fur, and entertainment. Many polls reflect the public's growing concern about animal welfare, yet most consumers don't see—or refuse to admit—that their behavior contributes to animal suffering. A 2013 poll by Faunalytics (formerly the Humane Research Council) found that 73 percent of adults surveyed believe people have an obligation to avoid harming all animals. So why aren't 73 percent of adults vegan? One reason may be that they haven't fully considered the issue of animal rights.

## What Are Animal Rights?

"Animal rights" can be viewed in two ways. The first is animal rights as a social movement to protect animals—even intervene and liberate them—from exploitation and abuse. The second is the idea that nonhuman animals, like human animals, have the right to be treated with respect as individuals with inherent value. Every animal is some*one*, not some*thing*, and they have the right to live free from humans inflicting pain and suffering on them. To deny this is to be guilty of speciesism, which is the idea that humans have been imbued with a set of exceptional attributes (such as speech, self-awareness, cognitive abilities, and a soul) that are unique to our species and thus give us moral priority over others. The animal rights philosophy does not place nonhuman animals above humans, but gives them equal consideration. This equal consideration means we should grant nonhuman animals the right to not be treated as objects—the same right we grant humans, at least in principle (more on that point in Chapter 3).

Of the many hurdles to affording animals rights, perhaps the trickiest is that animals are considered property, a legal status that does everything to ensure that the rights of the animal's "owner" are protected and next to nothing to protect the animal. Instead, the law presumes that owners of animals—farmed animals, animals used in research, animals used in entertainment, etc.—will recognize that it is in their economic interest to provide for their animals' welfare. So archaic is the concept of what constitutes animal welfare that the Model Penal Code, a statutory text drafted by the American Law Institute in 1962, defines the primary role of anticruelty laws as being to "prevent outrage to the sensibilities of the community," with the animal-cruelty provision categorized under "Offenses Against Public Order and Decency." Sounds like something from the eighteenth century.

Animal advocates are working to change that, but it's like turning a cruise ship. Actually, it's more like turning a cruise ship during a storm while it's capsizing amid a flotilla of battleships, each skippered by a captain with a vested interest in watching you sink. Fortunately for the animals, there are many determined people dedicated to righting the ship and moving it in the ethical direction.

## Animal Law

Because the law classifies nonhuman animals as property—commodities who can be bought and sold—they can be treated pretty much as their "owners" see fit. Even some of the most egregious examples of institutionalized animal abuse are tolerated under the law. Yes, we have animal protection laws, but they are notoriously weak and filled with loopholes. Under the Common Farming Exemptions that are enacted state by state in the US, for instance, it is at present perfectly legal for the egg industry to grind up live male chicks soon after they are hatched because it's considered the most expedient way to rid farmers of animals who are of no value to them, since they don't lay eggs. How can any reasonable person think this is humane treatment?

In light of such an impoverished ethos, some reformers work to advance the interests of animals through the legal system. Among these activists are attorneys specializing in animal law, a field of legal practice that emerged in the 1970s as a large-scale, organized movement in the United States and continues to make strides on behalf of animals. Numerous victories—from liberating a lonely bear from years of captivity in a roadside zoo to legislation affecting millions of farmed animals—are directly linked to the efforts of animal lawyers who participate in animal law programs at major universities. As the nonprofit Animal Legal Defense Fund (ALDF), one of the founders of the animal law movement, puts it, "We may be the only lawyers on Earth whose clients are all innocent." ALDF and advocates like it file lawsuits to protect animals and establish the concept of their legal rights, regardless of the species or the ownership interest of humans. They use courtrooms to challenge institutionalized forms of animal abuse and oppression. Animal rights cases have even been argued in the US Supreme Court.

## Legal Personhood

One way to gain protections for animals is to extend the definition (and rights) of personhood to certain species. This is not to say that animals would be considered *human*. That's a biological term that describes our species, while to call someone a *person* is to characterize what they inherently are: conscious and sentient.

Many people agree these traits apply to great apes—bonobos, chimpanzees, gorillas, and orangutans—and it's an important argument made by the Great Ape Project (GAP). Founded in 1993 by philosopher Paola Cavalieri and ethicist Peter Singer, author of *Animal Liberation*, GAP has been campaigning for the United Nations to adopt its Declaration on Great Apes, which extends to nonhuman apes the protection of three basic interests: the right to life, the protection of individual liberty, and the prohibition of torture. Once these rights are established, GAP would demand the release of great apes from captivity around the world.

The campaign has a global following. In 2007, the Balearic Islands, an autonomous part of Spain, passed the world's first legislation granting legal personhood rights to great apes. The concept is gaining traction elsewhere, including Argentina, India, Spain, Switzerland, and the US, the last of which is where animal law attorney Steven Wise has founded the Nonhuman Rights Project (NhRP). The NhRP argues that nonhuman animals who are scientifically proven to be self-aware, autonomous beings—such as great apes, elephants, dolphins, whales, and African gray parrots—should be recognized as legal persons under US common law, with the fundamental right to bodily liberty (the right not to be imprisoned in zoos, research labs, roadside menageries, etc.).

Wise's campaign for animal personhood is a response to his

frustration with welfare laws and regulations that have failed to keep animals out of abusive environments. Animals, he points out, currently have no more rights than a table or a toaster, so it's little wonder the law does nothing to protect them. "The example I give is that I can take a baseball bat and smash the window of your car, and I'll be charged with something," Wise said during a 2013 talk at George Washington University. "But the car or the windshield doesn't have legal rights. It's not a person. Essentially, a nonhuman animal is a kind of animate windshield. If I'm cruel to her, I can go to jail, but the nonhuman animal is a complete bystander to this. She doesn't have any rights."

Wise and his colleagues at the NhRP have filed numerous lawsuits on behalf of chimpanzees in captivity, arguing that personhood derives from cognitive and emotional qualities that these animals, like humans, possess in abundance. Chimps are extraordinarily complex, self-aware, and autonomous beings, says Wise, and they deserve their freedom. The NhRP is operating under the common law because they consider it more flexible than statutory law. Common law judges are supposed to take into account changing public morality and scientific under-standing and align laws to reflect them. As of this writing, none of the NhRP's suits has resulted in legal personhood for great apes, but it's only a start. And as more courts declare that nonhuman animals have autonomous lives to live, such ground-breaking institutional change will herald a major shift in public attitudes.

In the US, corporations have the same legal protections as humans—so why not animals? Probably because doing so would threaten the many ways we use our fellow creatures.

## Animals Used for Food

Of all the ways that humans take from other animals, turning them into food ingredients is likely the oldest—and laden with the most baggage. For most people, the act of eating meat, eggs, and dairy foods is their only contact with farmed animals, and it is often accompanied by a host of dining traditions and habits that make consuming them a comforting experience. This is what I mean by baggage. One of the principal reasons we cling to that habit of meat-eating is that it's a group ritual filled with emotional potency — transporting us back to a wonderful childhood memory in Grandma's kitchen, for example, barbecues with Dad, or enjoying a holiday meal in which a dead animal has always been the centerpiece. There are moments when I'm walking near a restaurant, smell a combination of black pepper, onion, rosemary, and sage, and am instantly carried back 40 years to Christmas dinners with my family. It's a powerful feeling.

It can be difficult to imagine a meal without animals. But that doesn't mean we have to eat them. Indeed, while demand for animal products is growing worldwide, in the United States, overall consumption of meat from cows, chickens, and fishes dropped 10 percent between 2004 and 2012, the most recent year for which the United States Department of Agriculture (USDA) has data. (The agency says US Americans are eating 25 percent less red meat.)

Being killed for food comprises many more cruelties than what awaits chickens, cows, pigs, and other animals at the slaughterhouse, and as we consider their rights, and a vegan ethic, it's important to at least briefly examine the relentless abuses animals suffer when they are literally born to become "food." This won't by any means be an exhaustive overview, but some of the common reasons activists agitate for farmed animals.

### Hens

Enter a typical egg-producing facility, as I have, and you'll find a windowless warehouse framing long rows of wire cages, often stacked five high. Some dim lightbulbs dangle from above, and you can see that each of these "battery" cages is occupied by six to eight gaunt-looking hens, each of whom has had the tip of her beak cut off so she can't peck her cage-mates. This painful mutilation also makes eating very difficult. The birds are packed so tightly into the cages that they can't even spread their wings. Other natural instincts, such as dust bathing and nesting, are but frustrating genetic memories for them. A huge pool below the cages collects chicken waste, and the ammonia from urine and the stench of manure burns your eyes and lungs. You can only imagine what the animals who pass their brief lives in this filth must suffer. Each hen has a tiny bit of wire area on which to stand, sleep, and lay her eggs. It's what she'll do day and night, producing at least six eggs a week for human consumption, until after about two years, her body depleted, she'll be pulled from the cage and killed, either at a "spent hen" slaughterhouse or by being gassed with carbon dioxide.

## Chickens

Of all the land animals raised for food worldwide, demand for chickens is by far the highest, due to their "efficiency" in turning feed into flesh and the few religious or cultural limitations to eating them. Chickens raised and killed for meat—called "broilers"—are bred in huge hatcheries and then "grown" in massive sheds. Modern farming methods have increased the chicken's growth to unconscionable levels, resulting in physical abnormalities. In the 1950s, it took 84 days to raise a five-pound chicken. Today—with agribusiness using selective breeding, special feed, and growth-promoting drugs—it takes just 45 days. Thus, most of the chicken's body grows rapidly, but the skeletal structure lags behind and cannot support the immense weight gain. Consequently, most broiler chickens have crippling leg disorders. They also commonly suffer lung problems and congestive heart failure. Just about all these abuses are suffered by turkeys and ducks, too.

## Pigs

One of the reasons many farmed animals are kept indoors can be exemplified by the domesticated pig. Factory-farmed pigs have been so genetically altered that they are extremely vulnerable to disease and must be confined in an artificial, pathogen-free environment. A bacterium that infects one pig could easily breach the immune system of another. So pigs destined for the meat case are kept in giant sheds. They stand with thousands of others on slated floors that allow their feces to squish through, and it all collects beneath them in massive pools, emitting poisonous hydrogen sulfide. Pigs, along with factory-farmed chickens and cows, are fed an assortment of antibiotics that fend off disease, pack on pounds, and give their flesh the pink hue considered appetizing to consumers. After three to six months, they are butchered. (The normal life span of a pig is 15 years.) The pig's mother will live longer, being artificially impregnated first at about seven months of age and then repeatedly to deliver piglets twice a year. She will exist in a perpetual cycle of pregnancy, birth, and nursing, her body first isolated in a tightly restrictive gestation crate until she is ready to deliver the piglets and then moved to an equally confining farrowing crate. She will go crazy from boredom and lack of mobility—she won't be able to take a free step and often can't even see her babies, who, at around 20 days old, are taken from their mother to be castrated and/or have a part of their tails removed without pain relief. Once she is considered "spent," mama, too, will be slaughtered.

## Cows

As the world's largest dairy producer, the United States accounts for some 15 percent of the planet's cow's milk, so let's use this country as an example. In 2012, the 9 million cows in the US dairy industry produced 200 billion pounds (90 billion kilograms) of milk. That is a staggering figure with a tragic backstory. In 1950, the nation's dairy farms had 22 million cows who produced 116 billion pounds (52.6 billion kilograms) of milk. To nearly double milk production 60 years later using 13 million fewer cows delights the dairy industry and makes them look like geniuses, but it requires some cruel calculus. It begins with moving most cows indoors and onto concrete floors, where each is tethered to a tie stall in which she cannot turn around or lie down comfortably. Some corporations house their cows on drylots, which are barren, crowded, and filled with feces. In either case, the US dairy industry has used selective breeding, drugs, and a genetically engineered bovine growth hormone manufactured by Monsanto known as rBGH (banned in many countries, including Australia, Canada, Japan, New Zealand, and the European Union), to transform cows into milk-producing mega-machines. As a result, cows' udders have become grossly distended, often drooping to the ground and becoming inflamed with mastitis, a painful and potentially fatal bacterial infection.

But arguably the biggest cruelty involved with milk production is one that even small farms offering organic or "humane" milk products can't avoid. To constantly lactate, the cow must deliver a baby, so the industry artificially inseminates her and then, once she gives birth to a calf she's carried for nine months, her baby is taken away so that her milk—milk that nature intended to nourish her calf—can be sold for human consumption. Cows form deep, enduring bonds with their babies, and this forced separation is a painful cycle she will suffer over and over until, after four or five years of "service" to the dairy industry, giving birth and producing 22,000 pounds of milk a year, her body will be "spent" and she'll be shipped to a slaughterhouse. Her male offspring, meanwhile, will either be killed for veal while still babies—after being chained for months in a wooden crate so they can't use their muscles and force-fed a milk replacement formula and antibiotics—or they will be fattened in the meat industry and killed for beef. Female calves face the same fate as their mothers: they will be raised on a milk substitute and go back into the dairy industry, where they, too, will be kept in confinement and will relive the heartache of being torn from their loved ones.

Their bovine cousins in the meat industry suffer the same separations, of course, and the calves raised for beef may be castrated, branded, and subjected to other excruciating mutilations, all without analgesics or anesthesia. One of the most traumatic standard procedures—done to cows in both the meat and dairy industries—is dehorning, in which the animals' horn tissue is burned out or gouged out of their heads with a caustic paste. Painkillers are rarely used. The industry claims hornless cows are safer for workers and other cows. Horns do serve an important function, however: they help regulate the animal's body temperature. Before the calves are a year old, they are sent to a crowded feedlot, where they receive an unnatural diet packed with antibiotics and growth hormones to quickly reach "market weight." The end for them comes when they are transported many miles without food or water to a slaughterhouse, where a harried worker holding a captive-bolt gun is supposed to render each cow insensible to pain with a shot to the head. But the lines move fast, and it never stops, so some terrified cows pass through fully conscious. They frantically bellow and flail as their throats are cut and they are shackled and hoisted on an overhead rail. Some former slaughterhouse workers say as many as 25 percent of cows die this way, completely aware of what's happening to them.

### *Fishes*

When it comes to animals used as food, fishes and other marine life seem to represent some unique category beyond the others. Even many consumers who call themselves vegetarian eat fishes, as if they grow on trees. Still others eat them believing that the industrialized consequences associated with the large-scale production of other animal products don't apply to fishes.

Living beneath the water's surface, with physical characteristics some find difficult to warm to, aquatic animals may be the most dismissed beings humans consume. They don't seem to vocalize. They don't have legs. They don't sleep. In fact, we know more about Mars than we do about most fish species, despite sharing a planet with them.

One thing we *do* know now is that fishes feel pain. Recent research has found that fishes not only have high sensory perception to process pain like other vertebrates, but they are very intelligent. They are also the animals humans eat more than any other, with the commercial fishing industry catching as many as 3 trillion fishes a year. (Many of these fishes are consumed indirectly, with about one-third of them ground up and fed to chickens, pigs, cows, or farm-raised fishes.)

Traditionally, most fishes were caught in the wild, either in nets by trawlers and dumped onto ships to suffocate, or impaled on one of the thousands of baited hooks on a long line, which may extend for 62 miles (100 kilometers). Because the procedure is indiscriminate, longline fishing is notorious for catching species far beyond what the seafood companies target, including dolphins, sharks, and endangered sea turtles. As much as half of what companies catch is dumped back into the oceans.

But as humanity's appetite for "seafood" increases, our oceans have been all but drained of fish populations, so a new industry—fish farming—has exploded. Also known as aquaculture, fish farming is now producing half of the world's fishes, all crammed fin to fin into marine or freshwater holding areas. Diseases flourish amid overstocked tanks and nets, so the fishes are given antibiotics, and cheap feed is provided in the form of pellets that contain the blood and bones of cows, sheep, and pigs, feathers from the billions of chickens slaughtered each year, as well as fishmeal and fish oil. Reproduction in fish farms is often performed using a process called "strip spawning." A hatchery worker pulls the female fish out of the water and uses his hand to express her eggs by applying pressure along the fish's abdomen, essentially squeezing the eggs out, like toothpaste from a tube, through the vent near her posterior and into a bucket or plastic bag. Fertilized eggs are later transferred to an incubator for hatching. Throughout the strip-spawning process, the fish is being manipulated and restrained, experiencing the trauma of suffocation before being plopped back into the water. For salmon and most other finfishes, death comes after their gills are slit open, sometimes following a blow to the head. Trout and Atlantic halibut, meanwhile, are killed by packing the animals on ice and letting them slowly suffocate, a technique meant to extend their shelf life.

Lobsters, crabs, shrimp, and prawns suffer a different sort of torture: they are commonly boiled alive. While I deplore animal studies, experiments show crustaceans such as crabs and lobsters do feel pain, making their lingering deaths in pots of scorching water especially cruel.

## Animals Used for Fashion

For those who live their values and adopt a vegan ethic, switching to an herbivorous diet is naturally followed by taking a close look at what's hanging in their closets. It makes perfect sense; after all, as we continue to embrace compassion, we want what goes *on* our bodies to be a reflection of what goes *in* them. For more and more people, caring about fashion means caring about the animals who suffer and die for leather, fur, wool, and ivory.

### *Leather*

Leather is the most common animal-based product people wear and carry, found in footwear, belts, jackets, bracelets, hats, dresses, gloves, skirts, watchbands, wallets, and car interiors. Meanwhile, from dog collars and leashes to horse saddles and stirrups, leather is affixed to animals we love—while it can be used to whip and beat others. Leather products are so varied in part because they involve the skin of so many species. Much of leather comes from cows, but it's also made from the skins of alligators, buffaloes, elephants, goats, horses, kangaroos, ostriches, sharks, sheep, and snakes. Contrary to the popular assumption, leather is not a byproduct of the meat industry but a highly profitable co-product. Indeed, some critics argue leather actually subsidizes factory farms, since sales of animal skins help keep meat prices down. But it's not only cows used for meat whose exploited bodies get turned into jackets and handbags: the leather industry also uses cows from the dairy industry.

### *Fur*

Humans have been wearing fur nearly as long as we've been eating animals. In fact, it was probably a *Homo erectus* hunter who became the first to drape an animal skin over his shoulders soon after consuming his prey. But what once might have been necessary for survival became obsolete with the evolution of fabrics made from plants and synthetic materials. Today, fur is a symbol of both extravagance and cruelty, with millions of animals being killed for a frivolous fashion accessory.

About 85 percent of the minks, foxes, rabbits, sables, raccoons, chinchillas, and other animals used for fur are raised and killed in fur farms, while the remaining furbearers are trapped in the wild. A typical fur farm is comprised of long rows of wire cages covered by a roof and surrounded by a fence. There might be as few as 100 or as many as 100,000 animals imprisoned within. Because animals have only been farmed for their fur for about 100 years, they remain genetically identical to their feral cousins. For them, freedom is a powerful biological imperative, so being held captive inside small wire boxes in fur farms literally drives them crazy. They react by engaging in abnormal behaviors, such as head weaving, pacing back and forth, twirling, and self-mutilation.

Trapping may be a distant second to fur farming, but there are still plenty of traps in the wild, especially in the United States, where trappers kill about 3 to 5 million animals a year for the fur trade—more than any other country. Not represented in this tally are "non-target" animals who happen to fall victim to traps, such as dogs, cats, and endangered species. The fur industry calls these animals "trash." The primary devices used to catch wild furbearers are the leghold trap, the body-grip trap, and the wire snare.

Whether they are trapped or farmed, these animals are killed in ways that do not damage their fur, including gassing, drowning, neck breaking, anal electrocution, suffocation, and poison injections.

## Wool

Of the animal products we wear, wool is the one that most consistently gets pulled over people's eyes—leaving the average consumer completely in the dark when it comes to the inherent cruelty of wool production. Like cows exploited for dairy, sheep used for wool suffer throughout their brief lives and are ultimately killed once their bodies have been exhausted. Some even die at the hands of impatient workers, who punch, kick, and even stab sheep with clippers during the shearing process. Moreover, to weaken the animals and make them less resistant to being shorn, they are denied food and water the day before shearing begins. Animal activists have witnessed such abuse on sheep farms in some of the biggest wool-producing countries, including Australia, England, and the United States.

One of the most disturbing practices in the Australian wool industry—the largest in the world—is called mulesing, which involves cutting a crescent-shaped slice of skin from each side of the lamb's buttock to produce a scar free of fleece, fecal and urine stains, and skin wrinkles. It's an attempt by farmers to eliminate incidence of flystrike—blowflies laying eggs in the feces that accumulates on the folded and excrement-trapping skin of Merino sheep. Flystrike causes pain, inflammation, and even death. What makes mulesing especially appalling is that through breeding, the industry has created the sheep to have abnormally folded skin (for more surface area to produce wool), making matters worse. Moreover, Merino sheep are not native to Australia and are easy prey for blowflies. Farmers deal with the problem the way they address so many other welfare issues: by mutilating the animals without any pain relief. Even sheep outside Australia endure mutilations. In the US, some 90 percent of lambs have their tails cut off to prevent feces from collecting in the wool.

Wherever they are bred and raised, however, sheep suffer in the wool industry. Shearing is supposed to be done in the spring as the weather warms, but some ranchers with large flocks begin the process too early in the season, leaving sheep without the insulation they need to survive cold temperatures. So if a sheep survives being beaten or stabbed by the shearing crews, he or she faces winter weather without any fleece. Some 1 million prematurely-shorn sheep succumb to exposure in Australia every year.

One of the dirty little secrets of animal agriculture is that sooner or later, every animal is killed. There is no retirement farm for wooly sheep, any more than there is for cows exploited for their milk or hens in the egg industry. (It's only a fortunate few who, by twists of fate, end up in farmed animal sanctuaries.) Sheep used for wool are killed once their fleece begins to thin out and they are no longer considered profitable. At age three or four—woefully short of their natural 20-year life span—the sheep are packed into a transport truck and driven to a slaughterhouse. In Australia, most "spent" sheep are loaded onto enormous vessels and shipped thousands of miles overseas to markets in the Middle East and North Africa, where they are ritually killed for both religious sacrifice and food. The voyage takes weeks, and each year, tens of thousands of sheep die en route due to heat stress, infections, and starvation.

## *Ivory*

Elephants have been under siege for their tusks for generations, with cultures throughout the West buying ivory products, but demand took off in the 1970s as newly affluent consumers in China and Japan propelled the trade to new heights. Ivory goes into the making of buttons, hairpins, pendants, bracelets, rings, earrings, and other fashion accessories, but it is most often used to produce chopsticks or more intricate status symbols, such as sculptures in China or traditional Japanese name stamps, called *hanko*, used in lieu of signatures on documents. One of the saddest uses I've seen is a souvenir elephant, complete with tusks, carved from ivory.

The ivory trade is part of a massive industry that traffics wildlife and their body parts, with tusks hacked from the faces of African elephants and smuggled to the far corners of the globe. In addition to the colossal cruelty involved, this illegal trade is responsible for an enormous financial transfer out of the poorest parts of Africa and into the pockets of organized crime syndicates, terrorists, warlords, and corrupt politicians.

Elephant poaching reached a tipping point in 2014: There are now more elephants being killed each year—nearly 35,000—than are being born. Conservationists say that if the demand for ivory does not abate, free-living elephants could be extinct by 2025.

## Animals Used for Experimentation

Because nonhuman animals share biological, physiological, and behavioral similarities with humans, the animal-testing industry regards them as the ideal tools for biomedical research, product testing, and education (such as medical and veterinary training). Researchers perform an experiment on, say, a rabbit or a mouse, and then extrapolate the results to predict the effects on a human being.

The use of animals as test subjects is one of the most contentious issues in the animal rights movement, with two sides facing off in a passionate debate. On one side are corporations, animal enterprises, and researchers, who claim that testing on animals is among the best ways to advance medical progress, develop treatments, and ensure product safety. Proponents also argue that there is no non-animal alternative to achieve cures and treatments, that experimentation is highly regulated, that animals are treated humanely, and that, because animals do not have rights, testing on them is acceptable. To gain the sympathy and support of progressive hearts and minds, they may even go so far as to characterize animal testing as a human rights issue, maintaining it's the ultimate use of animals for human benefit.

On the other side is a growing contingent of compassionate consumers and anti-vivisection activists—including scientists and medical doctors—who argue that animal testing has no place in modern society. They contend that even though *Homo sapiens* share certain parallels with other animals, nonhumans do not make good models for research. For instance, chimpanzees share 99 percent of their DNA with humans, yet AIDS researchers have given HIV to thousands of chimps without AIDS developing. The immune systems of the two species are simply different. Animal advocates would therefore agree with vivisection proponents that this is indeed a human rights issue, but only because animal tests do not reliably predict results in humans. Consider that 92 percent of drugs that prove safe and therapeutically effective in animals fail in clinical trials using humans, and that of the 8 percent of drugs that do pass clinical trials, more than half are found to have toxic or fatal effects that were not predicted by animal experiments. That's deeply troubling, to say the least. More efficacious and humane solutions include using *in vitro* studies on human cells and tissues, computers to model diseases, clinical research, and epidemiological studies (population studies) to examine the cause-and-effect relationship between lifestyle (such as diet, occupation, and habits) and disease.

But, more importantly, it's an animal rights issue. We have a moral obligation to protect the vulnerable, and this includes nonhuman animals, who have their own right not to be treated as a science project. In no vision of a peaceful future can I see a world in which we inflict torture upon animals in the name of human benefit—or for any other reason. As a reflection that the tide is slowly turning away from using animals, in 2015, the National Institutes of Health quietly ended the US government's longtime funding of experiments on chimpanzees, admitting that new scientific methods and technologies have rendered their use in research largely unnecessary.

Some countries have laws to protect animals in labs, but in reality they are no help to those who suffer. In the US, for example, animal testing is regulated by the federal Animal Welfare Act, which not only excludes birds, rats, mice, and cold-blooded animals—in other words, 95 percent of animals used for research—but only regulates the animals' housing and transportation, not the experiments they are used in. Those experiments can be carried out in any manner the researcher sees fit. Animals in labs are beaten, blown up, burned, and blinded. They are starved, suffocated, shaken, and shot. They are nailed down, tied up, and sliced open. Their organs are pulverized, their limbs are severed, their bodies are irradiated, and their spirits are broken. They are forced to inhale tobacco smoke, drink alcohol, and consume a variety of highly dangerous narcotics, including heroin.

Fortunately, countries are beginning to acknowledge that at least some animal testing is cruel and unnecessary. India, Israel, New Zealand, Norway, South Korea, and the entire European Union have banned the testing of cosmetics on animals, and other countries are sure to follow. With so many governments closing down cosmetics testing on animals, one has to wonder when the US is going to get on the "ban wagon."

## Animals Used for Entertainment

Using animals for entertainment goes back thousands of years, and it has never done anything more than benefit the oppressors and provide a few momentary thrills for spectators while condemning the animals to a life of confinement and extreme psychological agony. Nearly all the industries discussed here argue that there is educational merit in what they offer, but this claim is really a façade to justify captivity and breeding programs, particularly in the case of businesses that feature animals forced to do tricks.

### *Aquariums, Dolphinariums, and Marine Parks*

The concept of fish and marine mammal attractions seems so innocent: give the public a chance to see aquatic animals up close. Sometimes, as with SeaWorld, whales and dolphins will even perform tricks as a soundtrack of popular music blares over loudspeakers. But behind the splashy veneer is an alarming assortment of mistreatment, from food deprivation to tearing mothers from their babies. Visitors rarely witness overt cruelty in aquariums, dolphinariums, and marine parks, but it is an inherent element of animal captivity. Whales and dolphins are still routinely captured from the wild, for instance, and sentenced to a lifelong loss of liberty. These are highly intelligent, socially complex species, and in confinement they are prone to neurotic behaviors, such as swimming in endless circles.

Public aquariums first became popular in the nineteenth century, exhibiting marine and freshwater life in artificial habitats. As construction and water-filtration technology has improved, aquarium enclosures have gotten bigger, but they still cannot come close to approximating the biodiversity, tides, and freedom of living in the virtually unlimited space of the open ocean, and the animals suffer from boredom. Even the best-engineered tanks confuse the critical senses animals depend on in the wild, such as echolocation—the sonar-like system orcas and dolphins use to detect prey and navigate their world. Within the impoverished environment of the concrete box that is an aquarium, the animals' sonar calls bounce off walls. "The dolphin's life in a pool leads to a confusion of the entire sensory apparatus, which in turn causes in such a sensitive creature a derangement of mental balance and behavior," said renowned oceanographer and conservationist Jacques Cousteau.

Life for dolphins is bad in aquariums, but it gets considerably worse in dolphinariums—arenas in which these marine mammals are not only confined in chlorinated tanks lacking any stimulation, but are trained for public performances. Most of these dolphins are torn from their families in traumatic hunts such as those carried out each year in Taiji, Japan, and sold to the captivity industry. (It is now illegal to import a wild-caught dolphin into the United States, so the captive-bred dolphin business is thriving to meet demand.) Dolphins brought to or born in a dolphinarium or other marine park must learn to eat dead fishes. These are their nourishment and reward during training, a technique known as "operant conditioning." Those who don't respond well may not get fed—or worse, they may be beaten by an irritated handler.

Such mistreatment is also practiced in marine mammal theme parks, where dolphins are joined by orcas, sea lions, beluga whales, and other highly intelligent species to pass their lives in shallow tanks for the amusement of paying visitors. Like dolphinariums, marine parks generally offer the animals no environmental enrichment—such as rock formations or plant life—since doing so would obstruct the public's view. Perhaps worse, these animals are often torn from their social units in the wild. But even if marine mammals were born in captivity, it is nearly impossible for the industry to maintain family relationships, since animals are frequently sent to other parks. They'll even take calves away from their mothers, who bond for life with their offspring. Dolphins, orcas, sea lions, and beluga whales are hardwired to swim or migrate incredibly long distances, so being imprisoned is an especially cruel fate.

And it is mind-numbingly dull. Sentenced to a life of extreme monotony, orcas try to relieve their boredom by gnawing on metal gates separating pools or by chewing on the concrete tank walls. This leads to broken teeth and exposed dental pulp, so to prevent potentially fatal infections, marine park staff use a variable-speed drill to bore into the teeth and then flush out the soft tissue. This is all done without anesthesia. Clearly in pain, orcas squeal, shudder, and sink away from whoever is holding the drill.

## Circuses

Animals in circuses are a throwback to the days when people were drawn to seeing a traveling menagerie. Circus trains brought bears, elephants, alligators, great apes, big cats, and other wondrous animals to far-reaching parts of the landscape, allowing residents from even small towns to see these exotic species up close. But performing animals are as archaic as the human "curiosities" circuses once exploited alongside them.

Of course, bears don't ride tricycles in nature, any more than tigers jump through flaming hoops or elephants balance on balls. Animals are made to perform tricks like these using physical punishment, deprivation, fear, and submission. They are frequently beaten, kicked, stabbed, and whipped to make them obey. One of the most notorious cruelties is the use of a bullhook—a rod with a steel hook and sharp tip at one end, much like a fireplace poker. Circus employees apply various parts of the bullhook to an elephant's sensitive skin, tormenting them to perform. The bullhook is also wielded as a club, with circus workers inducing substantial pain by beating the animals on the head, face, legs, trunk, and back. To the extent that such assaults succeed in making a "wild" animal submissive, a part of that animal's spirit is destroyed. Such is the goal of "training" elephants, big cats, and other animals used in circuses.

Research on the welfare of animals traveling in circuses reveals that they spend 91 to 99 percent of their time confined in cages, carriers, or other enclosures that are typically one-quarter the size recommended for the same animals in zoos. That the space provided for animals in circuses is four times smaller than what they're given in zoos—and that they spend most of their lives like this—says more about humanity's animus toward our fellow creatures than just about any other cruelty we subject them to. It's little wonder that elephants, bears, big cats, and other animals are literally going insane under the Big Top, engaging in repetitive, neurotic behaviors, such as pacing in their cage, head-bobbing, over-grooming, and self-mutilation.

## Films and Television

I loved watching animal shows when I was a kid. *Flipper* and *Gentle Ben* were two of my favorites, and *The Wonderful World of Disney* frequently featured woodland critters interacting with humans. Even then I knew the animals were acting, but I had no idea how they suffered for filmed entertainment.

Most animals used in movies and television are born in captivity. For a wild animal, such as a chimpanzee or tiger, being denied nearly all their natural instincts has profound psychological consequences, and they exhibit this stress through the same kind of abnormal behaviors (pacing, over-grooming, etc.) animals in circuses exhibit. Once they've grown too big to handle or have outlived their usefulness for entertainment, animals are often sold to the pet trade or a roadside zoo, where they will languish behind bars.

Food deprivation is one of the tools of the trade for training animal actors, as are intimidation, electric prods, sticks, and fists. Indeed, fear plays a major role in making animals perform, and if you look closely, you can see it on the faces of great apes. Like the misleading "smile" of a dolphin—whose gently curved mouth creates the illusion they are always happy, even in a tiny tank—the "smile" of chimpanzees and orangutans is deceiving. When these primates bare their upper teeth, they are not happy; they are displaying what primatologists call a "fear grimace," which looks like a human smile. Just off camera near every "smiling" chimp in movies, in commercials, or on greeting cards is a trainer threatening to abuse him, so his fear grimace is understandable. (When chimpanzees are happy, incidentally, they show only their bottom teeth.)

You may be thinking, *Hold on. What about the "No animals were harmed..." disclaimer at the end of films?* Well, this certification from the American Humane Association (AHA) is virtually meaningless. AHA monitors animal and insect welfare in movies and television, but with its limited resources, it cannot possibly be on every set where an animal is used. Moreover, they are largely funded by a grant from the entertainment industry, so the movie business is essentially policing itself. In truth, animals are injured or killed during the making of films and TV shows all the time, and the producers frequently manage to earn the AHA certification provided the animals were not intentionally harmed or the incidents occurred while cameras weren't rolling.

Luckily, this form of exploitation may soon be extinct. As technology improves, more filmmakers are turning to special effects wizards to create lifelike, computer-generated animals who don't need to be trained and who always get it right on the first take.

### Zoos

From the outside looking in, it's easy to think of zoos as pretty decent places. It seems the animals are fed, they get veterinary care, and they live in neat little areas that simulate the real world. Some zoos do try to provide quality care, but even the best zoo is really just holding animals captive in an inadequate, artificial environment. How could a zoo in, say, Florida possibly satisfy the unique requirements of a polar bear? In fact, how can any zoo anywhere meet the needs of animals who in nature would be running, climbing, or flying; hunting or foraging; mating with partners of their choice; and otherwise living lives of freedom?

The fact that zoos call the animals "collections" and their animal habitats "exhibits" should tell you a lot about them. They profess to be about conservation and education, but zoos are, first and foremost, profit-driven enterprises built on a business model of capturing and trafficking animals, tearing them from their families and surroundings. As we consider human rights alongside animal rights, it's important to note that zoos are traditionally tied to colonialism, with invading nations taking the animals of foreign lands as the spoils of conquest and bringing them home to populate their zoological gardens. These empires weren't just grabbing gold or silver, they were appropriating a people's natural culture. It was the ideal way for imperial powers to inspire awe in their subjects and dread in those they subjugated.

Because they require a constant supply of animals, many zoos engage in captive breeding programs. These generate baby animals for zoos to display and bring in more visitors. Breeding programs are problematic in themselves, but they also result in "surplus" animals, who end up sold to roadside zoos, research labs, or to hunting ranches, where hunters choose from a menu of trophy species they're guaranteed to kill—there's no fair-chase ethic here. Sometimes the animals are butchered and fed to the zoo's big cats. Many animals are simply euthanized, a solution that has become ever more common in Europe. The Copenhagen Zoo, for example, kills 20 to 30 healthy animals every year—including giraffes, hippos, and even chimpanzees.

A common argument is that zoos perform an important role in society by educating the public. Survey after survey, however, tell us that zoo visitors show no indication of learning about animals or environmental conservation. One study showed that children even demonstrated a "negative learning outcome," with kids feeling they are unable to take "effective ameliorative action" on matters relating to conservation after their zoo experience. Kids are smart and intuitive. They know they don't need a zoo to learn about the animals they love. Consider dinosaurs. Children love them, and no zoo on Earth has a T-rex or Velociraptor in captivity.

Zoos were popularized as a way for urbanites to reconnect with nature, but actually they may be the perfect example of humanity's desire to master and control the natural world, a topic we will explore in Chapter 4. Zoo walls represent a dividing line between "us" and "them"; between intellect and instinct. We are separate from the animals, and therefore superior—or so we think. How tragic that visitors spend a few fleeting moments looking at an animal in a cage, while the animals are forced to spend a lifetime staring back.

To someone who sees no problem with eating or using animals I ask, *What quality about animals would make you stop? Their capacity to feel pain, sadness, and fear? Their ability to form bonds with others? Their intelligence? Their curiosity? Their desire to live?* Just like us, nonhuman animals possess all these.

Contrary to what some believe, exploiting animals does not help humans. Indeed, it robs us of the very element that makes us who we are: our humanity.

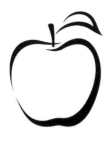

## Chapter 2

# On Veganism

*The food we eat masks so much cruelty.*
—Angela Davis

If we were to chart the modern evolution of veganism, our diagram might well depict something akin to the left side of Mt. Everest, with interest in this lifestyle that abstains from animal products climbing higher and higher over the years. Let's take Wikipedia as just one metric. In August 2008, the English Wikipedia article on veganism was viewed 21,536 times; in August 2013, it was viewed 145,358 times—an increase of nearly 700 percent. Of course, online interest does not necessarily translate into active participation, but as a barometer of how popular something is, it's tough to argue with those numbers.

One of the reasons for this increase can no doubt be attributed to the mounting evidence showing how much healthier plant-based foods are than animal-based foods. But, undeniably, a key factor in the popularity of veganism has also been the growing consciousness surrounding the use of animals. More and more consumers are not only turning away from eating meat, eggs, and dairy, but they are embracing a vegan ethic by boycotting marine parks, speaking out against animal testing, and rejecting clothes made of wool. By going vegan, we not only cease to financially support businesses that exploit animals, but we show compassion for ourselves as we reclaim our bodies and return to a more holistic diet.

Although the practice of eschewing meat, eggs, dairy, leather, and other animal products is not a new one—in 1813, for example, Percy Bysshe Shelley publicly objected to any food that came from an animal, and Amos Bronson Alcott founded what was essentially a vegan community in 1844—veganism came into its own in the twentieth century. In 1944, six non-dairy vegetarians gathered in England to discuss forming a new group. To describe their philosophy and lifestyle, they called themselves vegans. Thus was the humble beginning of The Vegan Society, which now has thousands of members worldwide.

Many people will say veganism is about giving something up. In fact, it's common for vegans to proclaim, "I gave up eating animals" or "I gave up meat, eggs, and dairy." While that may be technically true, it does not fairly represent what veganism is really all about, and it characterizes being vegan as some sort of dietary penance. Veganism is not really about giving up anything—it's about opening up to new things: new foods, new flavors, new friends. Yes, you're abstaining from meat, dairy, and eggs (as well as honey), but to focus on what you're *not* eating is to deny yourself the full pleasure of veganism while also sending the message that you're missing out on something. The only thing a vegan misses out on is contributing to the intentional killing of animals. Being vegan means you don't have to apologize to your food.

Donald Watson, one of the founders of The Vegan Society, put it this way in a 2002 interview: "In the early days our critics used to say, 'You don't know what you're missing!' We know now! We're missing an awful lot that they're having! Conditions so serious that it shortens their life by many decades, gives them pains and illnesses very soon after the first flush of youth has passed, and ties them to that medicated regime for the rest of their lives." This is one reason I tell people I'm vegan because it is a matter of life and death.

## It's More Than Food

Unlike people who embrace plant-based eating for their health, ethical vegans change more than just their diets. Of course, eating is a huge part of all our lives, so most of the vegan experience pertains directly to food. Indeed, most vegans love food. They blog about it; they trade recipes; they meditate on the virtues and vices of the latest nondairy cheese. When a new plant-based restaurant comes to town, you can count on vegans to patronize and promote it. Most of this chapter will be a discussion of food, but as we explored in the previous chapter, the exploitation of animals goes well beyond eating them, so it's important to consider what this means for a vegan ethic.

### *Clothing*

When it comes to leather, wool, and other clothing made from animals, new vegans do one of two things. They either get rid of it right away—perhaps donating the old clothing to a charity— or they wait until the shoes, belts, sweaters, etc., have worn out, at which point they look for vegan replacements. Fortunately, there are many companies that make high-quality vegan clothing, so there's no need to buy wool or leather to look stylish while staying comfortable. The technology to produce synthetic material that looks like leather has gotten so good that I cannot wear certain pairs of my shoes while engaged in activism, lest a passerby accuse me of being a hypocrite.

### *Medicines and Cosmetics*

Some vegans claim their lifestyles are so healthy they never get sick and therefore don't need medication and never see doctors. Well, good for them. For the rest of us, the issue of whether or not to take medicine isn't as simple as tossing out a leather belt or choosing beans over beef. Not only are animal ingredients commonly found in drugs, but most countries require that drugs pass a battery of cruel tests on animals before they can be prescribed. So even if we manage to find medications that don't contain gelatin or lactose or some other animal-derived component, we're still faced with a serious ethical dilemma.

One approach is to ask your pharmacist to refer you to a compounding pharmacy, where a pharmacist can create a particular medication without byproducts and dyes. (In the nineteenth century, prior to drugs being mass produced, pharmacy compounding was actually the norm.) This is an expensive option, but you'll find these specialist pharmacies in most large cities. You can also go the holistic route, seeking treatments that don't require drugs at all. For example, you might try physical therapy or acupuncture for shoulder pain, rather than a painkiller. I suffered for years with a pain in my legs (the result of some misadventure while traveling in Europe), but a chiropractor helped rid me of it.

Ultimately, of course, the choice is yours. Is it more important to remain steadfast and potentially be crippled by pain or possibly die, or to accept the regrettable truth that it's just not possible to avoid every single animal ingredient in our lives?

Unlike medicines, laws do not require cosmetics, shampoos, detergents, and other household products to be tested on animals—though they often are. To avoid supporting this cruelty, look on the product for a "Not tested on animals" label or for the popular Leaping Bunny logo before you buy.

### *Entertainment*

Fortunately, this one is easy. Ethical vegans do not knowingly patronize businesses that exploit animals. I say "knowingly patronize" because there's always a chance you'll buy a ticket for a theme park, and once inside discover they have animals. But most enterprises exploiting animals for entertainment are easy to recognize. These include circuses, zoos, marine parks, aquariums, and dolphinariums. Nor do vegans generally attend county fairs, which feature all kinds of farmed animals. And it goes without saying they would avoid rodeos, horse races, dog races, or other "sporting" events where the animals used for competition often die.

If boycotting these businesses makes it seem like vegans are too rigid and never have any fun, consider it from the animals' perspective. Their use for entertainment continues because people pay to see them being exploited. Moreover, it's because of those who speak up for animals that the captivity industry is making changes. Ringling Bros. and Barnum & Bailey Circus, for example, has stopped using elephants in its performances, thanks to activists and legislators campaigning against the use of the bullhook, and countries around the world, especially in Latin America, are shutting down their circuses with animals altogether.

## Going and Staying Vegan

Being vegan feels good. You're discovering new tastes, enjoying health benefits, not harming animals, and minimizing your impact on the planet. For many people, that's plenty of motivation to go and stay vegan. But others need a little more help. Maybe they're concerned about feeling deprived or they worry how their friends will react when they use the V-word at a restaurant for the first time. The main reason people do not go vegan is they think it's too difficult, so here's some advice for making the transition easier and sticking with it.

### *It's Not a Fad*

Veganism is often referred to as a "plant-based diet," so it's natural to think of it as some kind of weight-loss system, especially when you see stories of celebrities who shed pounds on a three-week "vegan cleanse." Most ethical vegans, however, will tell you it's not a diet, but a practice, a philosophy, a lifestyle, a political position, an ideology, or even a religion, since veganism relates to the profound truth that all life is sacred and connected. Not all vegans maintain their commitment, but those who go vegan for the animals are less likely to abandon their diet than those who do so for their health. It doesn't take an iron will to go vegan—just a willingness to try new things.

## Get Some Vegan Cookbooks

Like taking on any endeavor, going vegan means learning new skills, and cooking may be the most fundamental. Invest in a few vegan cookbooks that look good to you, or check some out of your local library (a few of my favorites are *Vegan Planet* by Robin Robertson, *Vegan with a Vengeance* by Isa Chandra Moskowitz, and *Eat Like You Give a Damn* by Michelle Schwegmann and Josh Hooten), then try at least one new recipe every week until you've got a wide variety of dishes you enjoy, including comfort foods. Not only will healthy meals nourish your body and spirit, but making a delicious dish for any non-vegan family and friends will show them how satisfying plant-based eating can be. A good vegan cookbook is much more than a collection of recipes—it's a roadmap to culinary adventures.

## Crowding Out

No one wants to feel like they're missing out on something, so try not to think of veganism as giving anything up (well, other than cruelty). Instead, gradually crowd out the animal-based foods you're used to eating with nutritious non-speciesist foods. The idea is to fill up on healthier choices first so that by the time you've given your body essential nutrients from veggies, legumes, and fruits, you'll have no appetite for unhealthy foods.

Some foods, like cow's milk and ice cream, are easily replaced with alternatives such as soy, rice, or nut milk. Replace meat at meal times with vegetables, legumes, and grains high in protein, such as kale, broccoli, spinach, potatoes, baked beans, lentils, rice, and quinoa. If you're really craving the taste of meat, try one of the many commercial analogues, like veggie meatballs or something from Tofurky or Field Roast. These so-called "mock meats" generally contain a lot of sodium, but they are delicious and satisfying for an occasional meal. And rather than reaching for a candy bar laced with milk or whey, grab an apple or an orange, which will fill you up without giving you a sugar crash an hour later.

As you taper off the animal-based foods and eat more of the healthy vegan foods, you'll feel satisfied and find yourself craving the unhealthy foods less and less. The variety of foods in your diet should actually expand rather than contract.

### Eat Whole Foods—Mostly, Anyway

I may be the last person who should be giving this advice, but eat whole foods. Whole foods are unprocessed, unrefined foods in their most natural state—the kind you'll find in the produce or bulk sections of your favorite market. As my friend Patti Breitman likes to say, to tell if it's a whole food, look at the ingredients; if it has any, it's not. Whole foods are your healthiest sources of protein, calcium, minerals, antioxidants, fiber, vitamins, and other nutrients. They are also packed with flavor. One of my favorite whole foods is steamed veggies with a bit of olive oil and nutritional yeast sprinkled on top.

But I have to be honest. There are just too many delicious vegan beers, onion rings, and desserts out there. I mean, have you *tried* vegan cheesecake? After all, we have to live a little, right? Yet even junk food without animal ingredients is still junk, so I try to keep it to a minimum. My breakfast is usually a kale-and-frozen-fruit smoothie, and I figure that's a pretty healthy start to my day. If I'm going to the gym before lunch, however, I sometimes take an energy bar with me.

Nevertheless, the common wisdom among vegan nutritionists is to consume whole foods. One way to help you eat more of them is to plan your meals for the week, then go to the market and load your cart with very fresh produce. If you're like me and you try to eat a lot of vegetables, you might find yourself going to the market two or even three times a week. Oh, and try to buy organic fruits and veggies whenever you can. These are better for your health and the health of the farm workers who pick them, since they are generally not sprayed with toxic chemicals.

## Dining Out

Some vegans are fortunate to live in places with plenty of plant-based restaurants. Living in, say, Berlin, New York City, or Glasgow, the challenge isn't so much finding a vegan restaurant as it is narrowing your choices to just one. But for every Portland or Austin or London, there are countless towns where the options are limited and disheartening. Thankfully, more vegan eateries are popping up all the time.

Given the choice, should we only patronize the vegan business, or is it OK to eat at a non-vegan restaurant? Everyone must solve this dilemma for themselves, of course, but I'll offer my opinion. I tend to hew toward spending my money at vegan places, since I want to reward them for not exploiting animals and help them succeed. But I also believe it's important to encourage other restaurants to offer plant-based meals—and thus demonstrate demand—so my wife and I also dine at places where veganism might not be their first priority. At a new Mediterranean restaurant near us, for example, lauren asked the owner if their hummus contained yogurt, explaining it would thus not be vegan. He then turned to one of his employees and said, "Never make our hummus with yogurt!"

## Practice Makes Progress

There's an old saying: Practice makes perfect. This may apply to learning a new language or mastering a musical instrument, but not to veganism, since there is no such thing as a perfect vegan. Nor should there be. Veganism is not a pledge of perfection; it is a promise to try your best.

Rather than struggling to be a "perfect" vegan—freaking out if you accidentally ingest an animal ingredient you hadn't heard of before—adopt the "practice makes progress" approach. Keep trying new recipes and share them with friends and family. Do all you can to avoid animal byproducts, but don't beat yourself up if you eat something by mistake.

Going vegan does not necessarily mean making the switch from an omnivorous to a plant-based diet overnight. Sure, some do, but for many people, it's a process. I, for example, took ten years to go from vegetarian to vegan, mainly because I didn't see any harm in consuming eggs. Like me, many people struggle to go vegan because they have a specific food they feel they can't live without. The big one seems to be cheese. To such people I ask, Can you stop consuming meat, eggs, and all dairy products except cheese (or whatever)—and then wean yourself off the cruelty by sampling some of the delicious vegan cheeses now available? Plant-based analogues for popular animal-based foods have come a long way.

Look at it this way. If you were embarking on a new exercise regimen, and you had a sore thumb, you wouldn't say, "Well, I guess I won't be exercising." No, because there are plenty of exercises you can do without impacting your thumb. So don't give up on migrating toward veganism simply because there's an animal-based food you think you can't part with. Once you try it, you'll find there are many fantastic plant-based foods to satisfy your cravings—including vegan cheeses!

Remember: Vegan isn't a station you arrive at. It's a way of traveling.

## Nutrition

This section is not intended to offer comprehensive nutritional advice—I would defer to a qualified vegan dietitian—but I do want to cover a few points and misconceptions about vegan nutrition.

## *Protein*

I often wear a shirt to the gym that says "VEGAN" across the front, and it occasionally inspires an interesting conversation. Not long ago, a guy at the drinking fountain squinted at my chest. "Vegan, huh?" he said. "Yes, that's right," I said. He furrowed his brow. "Where do you get your protein?" "From plants," I said, to which he scoffed, "Man, you need meat to build muscle and be strong." "Tell that to a gorilla," I said.

A common myth about a plant-based diet is that vegans don't get enough protein, which is an important building block of muscles, bones, cartilage, skin, and blood. First of all, humans don't need as much protein as popular culture—and people at the gym—would have us believe. It's recommended that vegans get 0.9 grams of protein per kilogram of healthy body weight (that's 0.4 grams per pound of body weight). So a vegan whose healthy weight is 170 pounds should get 68 grams of protein every day. This is no problem for most vegans, because there are many, many protein-rich legumes, vegetables, and grains. Eat a simple meal consisting of, say, one cup of cooked black beans (15.2 grams of protein), one cup of quinoa (8 grams), and two cups of cooked broccoli (10.4 grams), and you've consumed nearly 34 grams of protein—half of what's recommended for the day. Adding a scoop of vegan protein powder to a smoothie is also a convenient remedy for anyone worried about their intake.

## *Vitamin $B_{12}$*

Unlike protein, vegans often do not get enough vitamin $B_{12}$, which our bodies need for DNA production and to maintain nerve cells. There's a lot of discussion about $B_{12}$—where it comes from, why animals have it, if some plants can be a source, etc.—

so I am simply going to tell vegans this: *Take a $B_{12}$ supplement!* Visit VeganHealth.org or TheVeganRD.com for more information.

## Vitamin D

Your bones need vitamin D for proper calcium absorption. You can get vitamin D the way our ancestors did, from sunlight, but many people aren't outside enough, especially in the winter. In the early twentieth century, with a labor force working more and more indoors, vitamin D deficiency became a public health problem and led to cow's milk being fortified. Today the popular assumption is that dairy milk is a good natural source of vitamin D, but it's no better than any other food that's been fortified. In fact, plenty of soy, rice, and nut milks contain vitamin D. Vegans will want vitamin $D_2$, either in fortified foods or in supplementary form, as it is made from yeast. Vitamin $D_3$ typically comes from sheep's wool.

## Calcium

The dairy industry would love consumers to believe that cow's milk is their only source of calcium—a mineral we need for healthy bones and teeth—indeed, they spend a lot of money to make us think so. But the truth is, dark leafy green vegetables such as kale, spinach, watercress, and collard greens are also naturally calcium-rich foods, as are broccoli, legumes, almonds, and oranges. Fortified soymilk is another good option, but shake the carton before you use it, as calcium can settle at the bottom.

## Iron

Most of us associate iron with meat. But this essential mineral, which the body uses to make oxygen-carrying red blood cells from our lungs to our tissues, is also found in dark leafy greens, legumes, tofu, spirulina, nuts, seeds, and whole grains. Other sources include foods fortified with iron, such as cereals.

Plant foods only contain one of the two types of iron, nonheme, while animal-based foods contain nonheme and heme. The body absorbs heme iron a bit better than nonheme, so vegans need to make sure they are eating an assortment of iron-rich foods. Too little iron can lead to anemia, an iron deficiency characterized by fatigue, loss of appetite, pale skin, and low body temperature.

One way to dramatically boost iron absorption is to eat foods with vitamin C while consuming foods with iron. This combination has occurred culturally for generations, such as eating falafel with tomatoes, hummus with lemon juice, or bean-and-tomato soup. Nutritionists recommend at least 25 milligrams of vitamin C in the same meal with iron—an amount you'll get from one serving of broccoli, Brussels sprouts, cabbage, cauliflower, cabbage, sweet peppers, or tomatoes. You'll get twice that from citrus fruits and juices.

## Omega-3 Fatty Acids

Omnivores get most of their omega-3 fatty acids—which our bodies need to control blood clotting and build cell membranes in the brain—from fish and chicken eggs. Omega-3s are also found in a variety of vegan foods, though walnuts, ground flaxseed, flax oil, and chia seeds are probably your best natural sources. You can also take a vegan supplement.

## Soy Foods

Soy foods such as tofu are high in protein and have been enjoyed by generations of people in Asia. In the West, it's also heavily consumed as an ingredient in mock meats and non-dairy cheeses. But soy is the topic of much debate, mainly because of charges linking it to breast cancer. Some articles have quoted studies that showed soy can increase tumor growth at the cellular level, while other studies have determined soy may actually have a protective effect.

Much of the alarmist rhetoric about soy can be traced to the Weston A. Price Foundation (WAPF), which advocates diets rich in animal products. (Among their claims is that people with high cholesterol "live the longest.") Funded by the very businesses that are losing market share to vegan foods—including soy products, which now represent billions of dollars in annual revenue—WAPF has been campaigning against the "dark side of soy" for years, calling it "the next asbestos."

Don't be fooled by the hysteria surrounding soy. Vegan dietitians say a couple servings of soy each day are perfectly healthy. (One serving of soy equals 1 cup (236 grams) of soymilk, or ½ cup of tofu, tempeh, soybeans, or soy "meats.")

## Vegan on the Road

As any experienced vegan traveler will tell you, a little research before hitting the road will go a long way toward helping you find vegan-friendly restaurants. HappyCow.net, for example, lists and reviews veg eateries around the world, so I visit the site and print a list of local restaurants before heading to a new destination. (Those of you with smart phones can probably do this kind of research on the fly.) If you're in a city that doesn't seem to offer vegan fare, look for Chinese, Ethiopian, Italian, Mexican, or Thai restaurants, any of which will almost certainly be able to satisfy your hunger. Another option is to shop at a market offering fresh produce, bread, and other foods you don't have to prepare. And it's a good idea to travel with a compact can opener and eating utensils, just in case.

If you'll be taking a long flight or train trip, you'll need to pack some food to keep with you, as most airlines and railway companies are not prepared to accommodate vegans—if indeed they offer anything to eat at all. I recommend packing food that can tolerate travel, such as a large sandwich, robust fruit (like an apple or orange), nuts, carrots, dried fruits, and energy bars. There's also a number of vegan instant meals-in-a-cup, such as soups and noodle dishes (be sure to only buy the ones that do not require heating in a microwave); my experience is flight attendants and the staff in a train's dining car are happy to fill these with hot water. Peanut butter or hummus make a great snack, but beware that these may be considered a liquid and could be confiscated by airport security if the container is larger than 3.4 ounces (100 ml). Either buy the to-go packs or put them in small containers. I also travel with a collapsible bowl, a spoon, and some instant oatmeal—add some raisins and you've got a tasty meal.

## Alcohol

Many new vegans are shocked and perhaps more than a little saddened to learn that some alcohol contains animal-derived ingredients, including:

- Gelatin—a collagen made from bones, skin, and hooves. Gelatin is commonly used to attract tannins and reduce bitterness in wine during the fining process.
- Isinglass—a form of gelatin made from the swim bladders of fishes. Many beers and ales are cleared of impurities using isinglass.
- Egg whites—used in the fining process for wine.
- Chitin—a compound found in the shells of lobsters, crab, and shrimp. Another material used in the fining process for wine.
- Cochineal beetles—carmine and cochineal are pigments produced from scale insects of the species *Dactylopius coccus* and used as a colorant in drinks such as wine and the aperitif Campari. Sometimes identified as "Natural Red #4" on ingredient labels.

But take heart! There is no shortage of vegan booze. For a frequently updated list of beers, wines, and liquors free of animal suffering, visit Barnivore.com.

## Vegan and Animal Rights Activism

Once they recognize the impact of veganism, it's only natural that many vegans will want to share it with others. Reaching out to the public through leafleting, tabling, or other forms of activism is one way, but you can also make vegan entrées and desserts for your family and friends.

Sharing vegan food with others is fun. Animal activism, on the other hand—though enriching—is often challenging. Who among us enjoys standing outside a circus or slaughterhouse holding a protest sign? Activists aren't doing this because it's our way of having a good time. We do it because we're passionately committed to helping others. I regularly protest outside an amusement park that keeps animals in captivity, but I would much rather be spending my Saturday riding their rollercoasters; I just won't knowingly patronize a business that exploits animals.

Some governments, including Canada, England, Spain, and the US, brand certain animal liberation activism "domestic terrorism." The FBI even calls the animal rights movement "the number-one domestic terrorism threat," even though—unlike certain rightwing extremists—animal advocates have never murdered anyone.

The threat of being labeled a "terrorist" could dissuade people from engaging in activism, which is precisely what the National Cattlemen's Beef Association, Fur Commission USA, the National Association for Biomedical Research, United Egg Producers, the Alliance of Marine Mammal Parks & Aquariums, the American Veal Association, and a rogues gallery of other special-interest groups had in mind when they urged the US Congress to pass the Animal Enterprise Terrorism Act (AETA) in 2006. The Act, signed into law by President George W. Bush, prohibits any action that interferes with or causes an economic loss to an animal enterprise. But it is an unnecessary piece of legislation, since activism involving trespassing and property destruction is already illegal, and it certainly isn't going to deter actions by underground groups such as the Animal Liberation Front. It was therefore really just an attempt by those with an economic investment in exploiting animals to instill fear in activists and push the spotlight away from the atrocities they commit in factory farms, laboratories, tourist attractions, and fur farms.

Some civil rights attorneys have warned that activists could be prosecuted under the AETA if their activism financially hurts an animal enterprise, which could include a restaurant or institution that profits from animals. In other words, say these lawyers, you could be charged with terrorism for distributing vegan leaflets in front of a McDonald's or for organizing a boycott of a marine mammal park. But the AETA specifically excludes such "lawful economic disruption," and the chances of being arrested while leafleting or protesting are pretty slim.

What activists *are* being arrested for is videotaping inside farms and slaughterhouses. So-called "ag-gag" laws criminalize the act of capturing images of cruelty on film or video, which activists have used to both alert consumers to what goes on behind closed doors and, in many instances, get workers indicted for animal abuse. Unfortunately, because it's those caught on tape who have usually been prosecuted, low-level employees are arrested while the owners and managers—responsible for day-to-day operations and training—are considered blameless. It's a bit like a dentist treating your diseased tooth with anesthesia rather than a root canal; you feel better for a little while, but the problem still exists. In many ways, indicted workers are themselves victims of the same industrialized system that exploits animals. (We'll explore this more in Chapter 3.)

Ag-gag laws have been enacted in states throughout the US, and other countries have shown an interest in importing this method of suppressing transparency and accountability, though some legislators have rightly argued that passing such laws sends a message that the industry has something to hide. What's often missing from the debate is *why* activists and whistle-blowers are risking their own freedom to document animal suffering. As we explored earlier, animals endure unimaginable cruelties while being turned into food and other "products." Animal liberation activists willing to go undercover to expose this mistreatment are among those who believe that the offenses committed in animal enterprises are far worse than the act of recording them.

## Beyond Traditional Veganism

It wasn't long ago that being vegan was so fringe that many people weren't even sure how to pronounce it. Today, bestselling cookbooks are extolling the joys of kale, vegan restaurants are pleasing even the most ardent omnivores, and new plant-based foods are being offered in corner markets, so I'd say veganism has gone from the margins to mainstream—or pretty darned close. The past is prologue. We've become an economic power-house. Now it's time to look critically at where we're headed.

Sadly, we are so absorbed in agitating for the rights of nonhumans that we don't realize there are solutions in the foundations that speciesism shares with other forms of oppression. If to be vegan is to be compassionate, then a true vegan ethic extends compassion to all. If we are vegan because we do not want to benefit from the oppression of someone else, then it only makes sense that we will not want to participate in the oppression of anyone. This, I believe, is our moral imperative—a path to peace, equality, and human fulfillment that the pioneers of veganism championed long before we began using the term "intersectionality" to describe how different injustices are intertwined.

There's a saying in the movement: Animal rights are human

rights. It's used as a slogan on buttons, T-shirts, and stickers. A popular animal activist chant echoes this sentiment: "One Struggle, One Fight! Human Freedom, Animal Rights!" How often do the movement's everyday activities genuinely reflect this attitude? Not often enough, I'd say. Some animal groups are quite vocally against human beings; indeed, they have gained notoriety with such stunts as simulating sexual assaults against women as a way to make a point about animal exploitation, or they've used body shaming to promote veganism. Yet if we ever hope to unlock the interlocking systems of oppression, acknowledging that we can't effectively address one social justice issue without considering the others is the key.

If, as the animal rights movement argues, there is no moral distinction between human and nonhuman animals—if animal rights *are* human rights—then it makes sense that we should be working for the liberation of all species. The key to granting that liberation lies in the system of domination that oppresses animals as well as humans. In other words, speciesism is intrinsically linked to racism, sexism, heterosexism, ageism, anti-Semitism, classism, sizeism, ableism, and other forms of discrimination. Because these oppressions share the same roots, no society that tolerates discrimination based on someone's race, gender, religion, or other social category will ever reject the exploitation of nonhuman animals.

People of color, Indigenous peoples, feminists, peace activists, and others who fight for liberation and equality have been imploring us to *wake up* and grant everyone the respect and dignity we wish for ourselves. It's time we embrace a new paradigm for social justice.

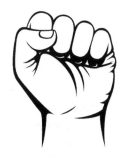

## Chapter 3

# On Human Rights

*Watch who they beat and who they eat.*
—Marge Piercy

According to some scholars, the entanglement of animal exploitation with other systems of oppression goes back perhaps 11,000 years or more, when foragers became farmers and began domesticating animals—herding them rather than hunting them. The theories of Friedrich Engels in particular have helped explain the origins of the patriarchal family, in which the wife becomes the head servant, the husband controls the household, and animals become private property to be handed down to male heirs. This theory helps explain how the domination of animals led us to dehumanize and oppress other populations; we had learned that the repression of animals expedited the repression of human beings. In both relationships, too, there is the under-standing—sometimes implicit, sometimes overt—that violence might be used to exert control.

I am not directly comparing any cruelties or disenfranchised groups; rather, I am suggesting that these are similar structures of subjugation with a common origin: patriarchy—men ruling over women and nature. A society is patriarchal to the extent that its laws, traditions, rituals, and customs revolve around men, and these men in turn dictate what role women will play in that society. The patriarchal ideology shares values with White supremacy, making it comparable to racism.

"Patriarchy" was not a word I heard growing up, but neither did I hear "middle class" or "White privilege," and I imagine that's because I was expected to assume these all applied to me, even if no one spoke of it. Now a universal ideology, patriarchy as a system has had consequences Neolithic cultures could not have possibly imagined.

## Patriarchy and Privilege

Patriarchy is an idea, and like any idea that becomes widespread, it has developed over time. In other words, the system we have now wasn't always the norm. What came before is a matter of conjecture. One view, embraced by some and rejected by others, is that in early human society, women held significant authority. Nineteenth-century anthropologists working in Europe interpreted evidence of goddess worship as an indication of matriarchal societies—egalitarian civilizations marked by peaceful cooperation and communal ownership and in which the mother was the head of the family, revered for her life-giving powers. Whatever the actual role of the woman in Neolithic society, with the advent of animal agriculture came economic surplus and the concept of personal possessions. The man became the "master of the house," dominating women, children, and the farmed animals—the origin of the term "animal husbandry."

Patriarchy was woven into the fabric of everyday life through religious customs, governmental structures, legal systems, and social values. Thus institutionalized, male dominance was literally king, though its structure is hierarchical: men typically have more power than women; men in the Global North have more power than men in the Global South; women of a more advantaged economic class have more power than men and women from a disadvantaged class; and people of color, children, the poor, the aged, and people with disabilities tend to be the most oppressed.

From such a social inequity, it's easy to see how discriminatory practices like racism and sexism could emerge alongside speciesism. But commonalities of oppression don't necessarily lead to alliances. After generations of Black people have been degraded by Whites calling them "animals," for example (some White soccer fans in Europe have even thrown bananas at Black players on the field), it is little wonder they would feel less inclined to consider animal rights when they themselves are still not seen as human. Likewise, while it's argued that animal advocacy is an inherent extension of feminism—with hens and cows being exploited for their eggs and milk, as well as both women's bodies and nonhuman animals' bodies being objectified as "things" (a "piece of meat") to be consumed—Joan Dunayer observes that feminists have historically rejected the animal rights cause because equating women with animals ("bitch," "cow," "chick," etc.) is seen as a way to dehumanize them. The sexist tactics used by some animal liberation groups haven't helped, either.

Breaking away from this latter tradition is the ecofeminist movement, which understands that dominance works best where there is disconnection and fragmentation. Consequently, this movement considers how feminism, racism, sexism, classism, colonialism, heteronormativity, and ableism intersect with speciesism: animal agriculture's exploitation of undocumented immigrant workers; the link between the bovine hormone rBGH and breast cancer; hunting as an attempt to conquer nature; the objectification of women in animal rights campaigns; veganism in relation to environmental justice; the myth of the "lab animal" as a willing sacrifice for the advancement of science; and many more.

In a patriarchal social system, no female—human or other animal—is seen as having ownership of her body. Those with power thus not only confine and manipulate other female species for human pleasure, but often deny full rights and freedom to others based on biases. Ecofeminists like Carol J. Adams, Greta Gaard, Lori Gruen, and pattrice jones argue that thinking holistically about how these and other forms of oppression interact can result in collaborative strategies for finding solutions. "Though sometimes called 'utopian' or 'concerned with too many issues,' ecofeminist theory exposes and opposes intersecting forces of oppression, showing how problematic it is when these issues are considered separate from one another," write Carol and Lori in their introduction to *Ecofeminism: Feminist Intersections with Other Animals and the Earth* (2014). "This approach also identifies the shortcomings with mainstream 'animal rights' treatments of speciesism."

Power can be demonstrated not only through patriarchy, but through privilege, which causes you to not acknowledge a problem, because the awareness of how you benefit from it is hidden from you. Privilege takes many forms: male privilege, gender privilege, White privilege, body privilege, economic privilege, English-speaking privilege, class privilege, healthy-eating privilege, education privilege, height privilege; society builds frameworks that bestow unfair advantages upon such groups, often unconsciously. Being male or White or tall or part of an advantaged class doesn't inherently make someone a villain—it's not what you are born with that matters, but what you do with it. Privileged people (myself included) take many things for granted, and overcoming privilege is especially challenging, since it is virtually invisible.

Reflecting critically on your privilege means confronting long-held assumptions and asking in what ways your behavior and consumer practices might be undermining the values you claim to hold dear. For instance, if you are White and are attempting to engage in vegan advocacy with a person of color, are you being sensitive to their unique cultural experience and identity? Don't assume that because you buy your produce at a farmer's market that everyone else has access to one. In fact, don't assume that someone else even *wants* to buy their food there. Likewise, just because someone doesn't match what our society wants us to believe is an "ideal" body type, don't assume they are an unhealthy eater. I could never possibly imagine what a Black woman living in a predominantly White community must experience every day as she navigates her world. But I can try to be respectful. I can listen more than I speak. I can remember that racism and sexism are real and pervasive and hurt everyone, regardless of their race or gender. I can let go of my ego and try to not get defensive when someone points out my privilege. I can recognize that working to benefit others does not mean helping one group become more like another group. And I can concede that I have a lot of learning to do and admit when I make mistakes—which is often.

Many vegan activists work on this issue, including Breeze Harper of Sistah Vegan Project, pattrice jones of VINE Sanctuary, and my wife, lauren Ornelas of Food Empowerment Project. I credit them for informing many of my views here, and I encourage you to seek out their writing, talks, and presentations. One of the important insights Breeze shared with me is that most White activists don't realize that their own whiteness is impeding their ability to be inclusive. "The challenge is to get them to understand that unless they pick up a book or go to a workshop that teaches them critical race literacy skills for a post-2000 age, they're probably not going to understand deeply what the problem is in terms of why their own work is not more inclusive or they're not on a path as an ally or building solidarity," she said. "No one who considers themselves to be liberal and a good person wants to hear they are part of the problem or that the work they are doing is not more inclusive."

Transformation is not easy, and one of the most difficult privileges that animal activists face is species privilege. I am not referring to the hierarchy humans exercise over nonhuman

animals—though this is clearly troubling for an animal libera-
tionist—but to an unintended consequence of speaking out for a
group that is not advocating on their own behalf. Though
animals do shriek, fight back, and make it clear in other ways that
they do not want to be exploited, animal activists are usually
their public voice, and we tend to project our own identities onto
the oppressed chickens, pigs, cows, fishes, rabbits, and other
animals. We empathize with them, recognizing that nonhuman
animals are the only beings who do not oppress anyone else yet
are in turn oppressed by members of all non-vegan social justice
groups. In this scenario, articulated by peace activist Andrea
Smith, animal advocates come to feel that *we* are the ones being
oppressed but not oppressing anyone else. This way of thinking
is toxic for building solidarity. We essentially absolve ourselves of
privilege responsibility and are prevented from engaging in
meaningful, unabashed alliances with other social justice
movements. As pattrice put it at an animal rights conference in
Washington, DC, "What you just have to remember is, no, you
are not a hen locked up in a battery cage. You are not a sow
locked up in a gestation crate. But you *are* a White person in a
country where people of color are locked up behind bars disproportionately."

When we consider our many privileges, we often overlook
access to healthy food, yet it's another way animal rights intersect
with human rights. In an effort to encourage ethical eating, some
vegans will say, "If I can do it, anyone can" or "Going vegan is so
easy." But such remarks are ill-considered. To begin with, having
access to cookbooks and information about veganism—even
Internet access—is a huge privilege, as is having the time to cook
plant-based foods. Even being able to *read* is a privilege. But
perhaps the biggest obstacle to veganism for many people,
especially those in communities of color and/or low-income
areas, is that they have trouble finding healthy produce in local
markets that primarily sell alcohol and snacks, which is where

they're often forced to shop. These markets may be poorly stocked with fresh fruits and vegetables, requiring residents who want healthy food to travel long distances to a grocery store— something not everyone can manage, particularly someone with a limited budget working late hours and relying on public transportation. On top of all these hurdles, vegan food can be expensive. As a result, it's often more cost-effective and convenient for them to feed their families a fast-food meal.

"This is a global problem," says lauren Ornelas. "It's a problem for First Nation peoples in Canada. It's a problem for the Maori of New Zealand. And it's a problem for communities of color, especially Blacks and Latinos, in the United States. This is a huge issue when you talk about veganism in these communities. People say, 'Why don't we have more people of color in the animal rights movement?' To talk to these people about vegan foods when they don't even have access to fresh fruits and vegetables is offensive. This lack of access is a form of food oppression. It's food apartheid."

## Human Rights and the "Cruelty-Free" Myth

Healthy food is central to everyone's quality of life, and access to it should be a right, not a privilege. But it doesn't end there. If the food we put on our plate is at the core of a vegan ethic, we have to acknowledge it's often wrapped in inequities that devalue and harm humans. Farm workers, children, Indigenous peoples, and individuals forced into slavery are among those whose basic rights are disregarded in an institutionalized hierarchy that largely favors White men. These people are also commonly subjected to extreme violence. So it's time we rectify the myth that if something doesn't contain animal ingredients, it is absolutely not the product of oppression. Eating would be a much more compassionate practice if this were so, but as lauren often says, "vegan" does not necessarily mean cruelty-free.

## Farm Workers

Unless you grow all your own fruits, vegetables, legumes, and grains, you owe a big debt of gratitude to the people who toil in agricultural fields around the world. Of course, growing one's own food used to be common, but today we import most of what we eat. The coffee you drank this morning could have come from beans grown in Vietnam or Colombia, while the banana you sliced onto your cereal might have been in Central America last week. Brazil is the world's biggest producer of orange juice and sugar, and India is the number-one exporter of rice. If you like carrots, you can thank the farm workers of China and Russia (the US is the third-largest producer). It's because of this global system that even produce with a short growing season is available in your grocery store year-round.

Regardless of where the food comes from, it's generally the result of grueling labor conditions for the men, women, and children who manually plant, cultivate, harvest, and pack fruits and vegetables. These are now frequently displaced small-scale farmers from the Global South, who travel to Australia, Canada, the European Union, the United States, and elsewhere in search of employment. They struggle to scratch out a living amid fields of toxic agricultural chemicals, employer harassment, and often extreme temperatures. Already among the most disadvantaged groups anywhere, migrant and seasonal farm workers—that is, those who move from one location to another in search of agricultural work and those who perform seasonal farm work in their local area—face harsh living conditions, low pay, and backbreaking labor. Adding injury to insult, without adequate legal rights, farm workers engage in one of the world's most dangerous occupations.

In addition to laboring outside in heat that can be fatal, workers cope with lacerations, respiratory diseases, melanoma, and noise-related hearing loss. On non-organic farms (and even some organic ones), they are exposed to agricultural chemicals, as pesticides, arsenic compounds, synthetic fertilizers, solvents, and other toxic substances are liberally used in the production of conventional fruits and veggies. The potential long-term, chronic effects of coming into contact with these chemicals include prostate cancer, non-Hodgkin's lymphoma, leukemia, neurological deficits, fertility problems, and passing on serious birth defects. Is it any wonder, then, that the average life expectancy of a farm worker in the US is only 49 years? That was the life expectancy for just about everyone else in the country in 1903.

Perhaps the most insidious danger is the persistent menace of sexual harassment and physical violence that female laborers face. Sexual predators regard undocumented women as "perfect victims" because they are isolated, often do not know their rights, and lack legal status. Perpetrators routinely taunt their victims with suggestive comments and degrading insults, gradually escalating to sexual assault. Spanish-speaking female farm workers refer to the fields as the *fils de calzón*—"fields of panties." While research on the extent of sexual harassment of workers is scant, anecdotal evidence suggests that it is rampant. According to one of the rare studies, done in California, nearly 40 percent of female farm workers said they had been sexually harassed. In virtually every case, the men held positions of power over the women, who often don't report assaults because of shame, fear of deportation or losing a job, language barriers, and unfamiliarity with workplace laws.

These assaults generally begin well before women enter the United States from Mexico. During a visit to a farm worker labor camp organized for Food Empowerment Project volunteers by Dr. Ann Lopez of the Center for Farmworker Families, we met a woman who had been sexually assaulted on her crossing to the US and gave birth to a son as a result. We learned that the fear of being raped by guides, fellow immigrants, criminal gangs, and government officials is so pervasive that many women now take contraceptives during their journey north. By one estimate, 80 percent of women and girls making the trek from Central America and Mexico in search of a better life in the US are victims of sexual violence.

Not long ago, lauren gave a presentation on this issue in Portland, Oregon, and the following morning we drove to nearby Eugene, where a number of social justice groups, including the Pineros y Campesinos Unidos del Noroeste (Northwest Treeplanters and Farmworkers United)—commonly referred to as PCUN—had asked her to give a talk on food justice in the evening. We visited the PCUN service center for farm worker families, taking to heart how the challenges for these workers always seem to be the same; only the crops they harvest change. Hungry for lunch, we were thrilled to find an all-vegan diner called the Cornbread Café, and settled into one of the booths toward the back. After ordering, lauren and I fell into a conversation about her presentation, and I asked her how consumers can help farm workers. "We can help by supporting regulatory changes, legislation, and corporate campaigns that encourage produce buyers to pay more for the fruits and vegetables they sell to consumers," she said. "These bring farm workers closer to earning a living wage. Also, we need to show the growers and policy makers that we want farm workers not only to make a living wage, but to be treated with dignity and respect in the fields. This isn't an issue that we can only fix by buying certain foods. We need to join our voices with theirs to help create fundamental changes in how they are treated."

## *Children*

Because of a loophole in United States labor laws, children of any age can work in the fields alongside their mother or father. And with the consent of a parent, kids may work on any farm from age 12 (although Human Rights Watch has interviewed farm workers as young as seven). After age 16, they are allowed to do agricultural work that the US Department of Labor deems "particularly hazardous" for children, such as using sharp tools or driving a tractor. These young people comprise one of the most vulnerable and least visible labor forces in the country. When most kids their age are in school, they are putting in 10- to 12-hour workdays, six or seven days a week.

Such treatment sounds like something out of a Dickens novel from the nineteenth century. As much as we like to believe that we live in a more enlightened age, children worldwide are exploited as a workforce—60 percent of them, or about 100 million, in agriculture. (This figure does not include the sex trade.) Some adults may not see a problem with kids working on farms, arguing that a little physical exertion in the fresh air "builds character." But this is not a small family farm we're talking about. In the US, most farms are owned by corporations, not families, and they require workers to operate heavy machinery and spray crops with highly toxic chemicals.

Toiling in severe heat, kids on farms prepare the land, transport and plant seedlings, apply fertilizers, spray pesticides, harvest, weed, and process collected crops. This is one of the three most dangerous industries (along with construction and mining) in which young people work around the globe; they suffer fatalities, injuries, accidents, occupational diseases, and other health consequences. Nearly 300 children are killed and another 24,000 are injured every year on US farms alone. Girls working on farms are also exceptionally vulnerable to sexual abuse.

No child wants to be exposed to the extreme hazards of agriculture. Depending on where in the world they are, there's a variety of factors that force children into farm labor, including poverty, a breakdown of the family, household shocks due to HIV and other causes, or family indebtedness. Many are children of migrant workers, and they live an itinerant existence moving with the seasons. All the while they are missing out on many of the benefits that should be a right of childhood, not the least of which are a safe environment and a formal education.

Again, consumers can help by supporting regulation, legislation, and corporate campaigns.

## Indigenous Peoples

Two of the most ubiquitous foods in the world—soybeans and palm oil—are slowly but surely choking off Indigenous communities by destroying their surroundings or simply displacing them from their lands. Soybeans are turned into tofu and other vegan products, of course, but 85 percent of soy is processed into meal and vegetable oil, and almost all of that is fed to farmed animals. It is also used to make biofuel, as is palm oil, which comes from a reddish, plum-sized crop that long ago surpassed the humble banana as the world's bestselling fruit. By some estimates, half of all household goods are made from palm ingredients, including such disparate products as margarines, lipsticks, pet foods, cookies, candles, peanut butters, and detergents.

Soy and palm are both monoculture crops, meaning they are the only plant cultivated in a given area for many successive years. The areas are often rainforests that have been denuded of all signs of life, thus ridding them of both their native vegetation and animal inhabitants, including the local human population. Soy and palm crops are then doused with pesticides that contaminate the soil and water.

With their subsistence-based ways of living, Indigenous peoples rely heavily on the environment, which the industrialized production of soy and palm quickly transforms into a vast wasteland. The tropical island of Borneo, to offer just one example, has been so relentlessly burned, bulldozed, and logged for palm farming that unruly rainforests are rapidly giving way to a landscape of neatly planted oil palm trees. Here, humans and other animals disappear in tandem as biodiverse peat swamps are set ablaze to create still more cropland and feed the ecocide machine.

All this destruction comes at a steep cost, and Indigenous peoples get stuck with the bill, which includes land disputes, violent conflicts, and even murders carried out on behalf of palm oil barons. As a result, greedy governments are handing over millions of acres in Indonesia, Malaysia, and elsewhere to palm oil interests, who then evict the communities living there. Implicated in the controversy are agriculture giants like Archer Daniels Midland, Cargill, and Monsanto, which have had to face tough questions about human rights violations in their palm oil supply chain. One of the most notorious examples occurred in 2011, when Indonesian police, allegedly contracted by Wilmar—the world's largest palm-oil processing company and one of Cargill's suppliers—ejected 83 families from three Sumatran settlements at gunpoint, then destroyed their homes.

Such confrontations ignore the rights of local inhabitants to Free, Prior, and Informed Consent, which has been enshrined in the UN's United Declaration on the Rights of Indigenous Peoples. People in many communities say the first they knew about a proposed plantation was when the bulldozers arrived. Lacking official land titles, local communities are frequently left with no choice but to accept oil palm farming. Even more troubling are stories of security forces on palm oil payrolls storming into villages and killing Indigenous peoples, many of whom have refused to relinquish their land. Human rights organizations and media outlets alike have reported such murders in Colombia, Guatemala, Honduras, Indonesia, and the Philippines. Rahmat Ajiguna, delegate of a 2012 international fact-finding mission investigating complaints of land grabbing, says that in 2011, Indonesian state authorities murdered 22 people involved in land struggles with palm oil companies: "When they resisted, they were killed."

Similar reports have come out of Brazil and Paraguay, where soybean production gives local inhabitants its own brand of social conflict. It has become distressingly common for small-scale farmers to be killed or injured as soy corporations move them off land in Paraguay, which since industrialized soy farming was introduced in the 1970s has become one of the biggest producers of the crop and where the "soybean war" has ignited into a national scandal.

Paraguay's neighbor Brazil is home to the largest expanse of Amazonian rainforest—some 2 million square miles (about 5 million square kilometers)—and it's gradually being torn apart tree limb by tree limb for soy plantations and range land while traditional forest communities and rural activists fight to preserve their tribal terrains. According to a BBC report, 833 Indigenous people were murdered in Brazil between 2007 and 2013, and many of these were victims of gunmen hired by soy tycoons who in turn are backed by a powerful agribusiness lobby. Local and national Brazilian authorities say they want to protect the Amazon and its inhabitants, yet they are seduced by the tremendous economic value of soy, which was introduced in the country in the 1990s.

Because of our concern about the effects of palm oil production on humans, other animals, and the planet, lauren and I avoid this ingredient in the products we consume. And because most of the human rights abuses associated with soy are in the mass production of genetically modified soybeans, we only buy organic tofu, which is generally free of GMOs.

## Slavery

Using humans as a source of forced labor to produce food and other agricultural products has a long and sordid history. Perhaps more shameful than slavery's indefensible legacy, however, is that it's still going on; indeed, there are more slaves today than ever before—as many as 30 million—despite the practice being illegal in every country. Most of these people are enslaved for manual labor in industries such as farming, ranching, and fishing. But millions of women and children are also trafficked for the sex trade (an issue we'll examine shortly).

Victims of forced labor are often tricked into taking a job with the promise of good pay in another country—pay that never materializes. Instead, the person's passport is confiscated and he or she is made to work under the threat of violence. Others are victims of bonded labor as a means to repay recruitment fees and the cost of getting them across a nation's border. Coerced or trapped into service, they work for very little or no money while the "debt" invariably grows and may even be passed on to a succeeding generation. In Nepal, for example, landless farm workers known as *haliyas* ("one who plows") are born into slavery because their ancestors borrowed from a landowner and were unable to pay off the debt. This system flourishes even though it has been officially abolished.

From involuntary servitude on fishing trawlers in the Pacific (where the sick are thrown overboard and the defiant are beheaded) to clearing forests for pastureland in South America, slaves are a no-cost resource for a corrupt food system. In 2015, US authorities busted a slave-labor ring that promised families in Guatemala a good life and education for their children. The kids were then smuggled into the United States, where they were forced to work 12 hours a day, seven days a week at Ohio egg farms. They received no pay, and those who refused to work were threatened with their lives.

Elsewhere in North America, thousands of laborers harvesting produce receive no regular pay, are fettered in chains at night, and share derelict lodgings—typically a trailer—with a dozen or more other pickers. Seven days a week they work fields surrounded by barbed wire. They are watched by armed guards. They are beaten if they try to escape. Some manage to get away, and sometimes authorities shut down an operation. But another one replaces it, and contractors fill the fields with slaves.

Much of this dynamic is the result of the downward pressure

placed on wages by enormous supermarket chains. By leveraging their tremendous buying power, they can bully produce growers into selling fruits and vegetables at preposterously low prices, which trickles down to what farmers can afford to pay pickers. When the consuming public thinks they're getting a great deal on tomatoes, little do they know it comes at the cost of freedom and dignity for those forced to harvest them.

On farms along the southern shore of Western Africa, meanwhile, slavery also taints one of our most popular culinary luxuries: chocolate. Plantations in Ghana and Côte d'Ivoire, accounting for 60 percent of the world's cocoa beans, are notorious for using the worst forms of child labor, which the International Labor Organization defines as including all forms of slavery, child trafficking, child soldiers, commercial sexual exploitation, hazardous child labor, and using children in illicit activities. According to Food Empowerment Project, children as young as five are trafficked from neighboring countries to work on cocoa farms, where they perform dangerous tasks such as harvesting pods with machetes, clearing land with chainsaws, and spraying crops with pesticides. Kids are locked in at night, and if they try to escape, they are severely beaten. Some are never seen again.

Forced labor and cocoa production have gone hand in hand since the first commercial production of chocolate in the nineteenth century, when slaves were taken from Angola to work the new cocoa estates on the island of São Tome and Principe, off the west coast of Africa. It seems nothing has changed except the location. With cocoa farmers in Ghana and Côte d'Ivoire earning less than US$2 a day—well below poverty level—resorting to the use of child labor is common.

The issue of slavery in cocoa production is one of the many injustices Food Empowerment Project focuses on, and rather than suggesting that anyone give up eating chocolate, their advice for now is to just be smarter about what you buy. To that end, their website (foodispower.org) features a frequently updated list of vegan chocolate produced without using cocoa sourced from areas in Western Africa where child slavery is the most pervasive. From the farmers and traffickers to the governments and multinational chocolate companies, almost no one in the cocoa supply chain acknowledges his or her role in enslaving humans. But as consumers, the least we can do is not support this cruelty with our wallets. Food Empowerment Project also encourages consumers to urge companies to be transparent about where they source their cocoa from.

## Slaughterhouse Workers

Let's be clear: No one wants to work on a slaughter line killing animals eight hours a day. It is grueling, violent, dangerous, and repetitive—all for a pittance in wages. Everyone I've ever talked to about this work speaks of it with disdain. One former Tyson chicken plant worker I interviewed told me that the management refused to halt the kill line, even to allow someone to take a pee. So, he said, "the workers were actually urinating right on the equipment—on the poles and beneath the live-hanging conveyor belt that brought the birds in from outside." Likewise, it's not uncommon for slaughterhouse workers to defecate in their pants.

According to Human Rights Watch, there are "systematic human rights violations embedded in meat and poultry industry employment." Workers suffer preventable injuries that are often severe and sometimes fatal. Moreover, as a consequence of killing animals, they experience a number of psychological issues that mimic the symptoms of post-traumatic stress disorder, including drug and alcohol abuse, depression, anxiety, paranoia, disassociation, and recurring dreams of violent acts. Simply put, abattoir workers cannot care about the animals they kill—or at least not exhibit any compassion they may feel.

Such abuses are embedded into the system, says Human

Rights Watch, because any meat company trying to respect the rights of its workers would incur additional costs and be undercut by competitive businesses.

Not only is this one of the most hazardous industries in the world, but meatpacking plants are fear factories in which its impoverished-immigrant workforce dare not speak up lest they run the risk of losing their jobs or being deported. Most of these people are economic refugees—pushed out of their home countries in a desperate search for employment—and they do not understand they usually have rights, such as workers' compensation benefits to cover work-related injuries in the United States.

For all these reasons, undercover investigations that publicly shame low-level slaughterhouse workers who abuse animals have little or no positive impact. They might make outraged members of the community feel an injustice has been remedied, but celebrating the arrest of a few underpaid, stressed-out laborers (typically people of color) only serves to reinforce the system of oppression by victimizing another disenfranchised group. Sometimes these employees are not even charged with animal cruelty but with possessing a false identity (used to secure work at the slaughterhouse).

I suggest we vilify the industry, not the individual worker. Yes, I too am sickened when I see videos that depict slaughter-house employees taking out their anger and frustration on animals, and I am not defending their actions. But we have to remember that the psychic weight of working in an abattoir takes a devastating emotional toll. Rather than attack the low-wage worker—who is always the one caught on video—let's pursue the structural perpetrators who are responsible for orchestrating an atmosphere of violence. If we are going to truly embrace compassion toward all, having empathy for slaughterhouse workers surely ranks as among our most challenging goals.

Of course, we can also acknowledge the role consuming animals plays in contributing to these abuses. The popularity of meat, after all, creates a demand for slaughterhouses and their dirty business.

## Partners in Crime

Because they are inevitably desensitized to suffering, many slaughterhouse workers have a higher propensity for aggression, and it doesn't end when they clock out for the night. They bring this anger home, which is just one example of how victimization can get transferred from animals to humans. But domestic violence and other crimes targeting women, children, and men are not only committed by people who witness or participate in thousands of animal deaths each week. Animal abuse has long been recognized as a signature pathology of history's most violent offenders, and law enforcement profilers now routinely refer to animal cruelty reports as they work to predict antisocial behavior.

In households, abusive partners frequently injure or kill the animal companions of their human victims—or threaten to—as a way to punish, inflict terror, and exert power. (Exacerbating this scenario, domestic violence shelters frequently do not allow animals, so battered women who escape their abusers face the choice of leaving their nonhuman companions behind or remaining at home to be further victimized.) Children growing up in homes with animal abuse and domestic violence often learn that such deviant behavior is the norm and pass these values along to their own kids, perpetuating the cycle of cruelty onto another generation.

Violence against humans and other animals is often showcased side by side in our culture. Depictions of women as "pieces of meat," for example, are echoed in similar images of dead farmed animals, such as chickens and pigs, arranged to remind consumers of sexualized human females, a theme Carol J. Adams documents in *The Sexual Politics of Meat*. As photographed or illustrated for meat industry ads, the dead animals are sometimes even portrayed wearing lipstick or high heels or their corpses are posed in a provocative manner. This type of marketing is meant to be clever, but it's clearly gendered violence that capitalizes on the oppression of two devalued groups. It conveys the unmistakable message that both nonhuman animals and women are objects to be consumed.

But intimate-partner violence can be intersectional in other ways. Consider the Black woman with a disability who is victimized by her same-sex partner, in which case her identities as a person of color, a lesbian, and a disabled person—all traditionally marginalized in mainstream culture—overlap. Author and activist Suzanne Pharr has noted that battered-women's programs that wish to work with battered lesbians must understand that it's not safe for these women to participate if the program does not discuss lesbians in its literature and public outreach. We can expand that concern to involve other social identities, including poverty. Many battered women who seek safety from abusive partners are unemployed or underemployed. Kimberlé Crenshaw observes that shelters serving these women must confront not only the violence inflicted by the batterer, but the many other systems of domination that often converge in these women's lives and prevent them from creating alternatives to abusive relationships.

It wasn't until 2013, when I heard pattrice jones speak at an animal rights conference in Luxembourg, that I learned of Crenshaw's work and gained a deeper appreciation for solidarity among movements. In introducing the topic of intersectionality, pattrice asked the audience, "What is 6 times 7?" A few people yelled out, "42!" pattrice said, "OK, everybody imagine 42. Now, what is the 6 and what is the 7? You can't say, can you? No, because the 42 is the product of the 6 and the 7 in interaction with one another." In a similar way, she said, Crenshaw used the term "intersectionality" to try to explain the relationship between racism and sexism. Though it began by addressing race and gender, intersectionality has gone on to examine multiple dimensions of inequity among other social categories.

## Other Types of Human Rights Abuses

A vegan ethic, I believe, should regard all exploitation and injustice as inexcusable—not just those that relate to food or animals. And while I can't possibly examine all human rights abuses to the depth they deserve, I do want to highlight several as examples. The prison industrial complex, for instance, is cause for considerable concern, and not only because some activists may be prosecuted for defending animals. Having long ago jettisoned any pretext as facilities of "rehabilitation" or "correction," prisons have become privately run institutions in which mass imprisonment is a form of discrimination. Indeed, there are now more Black men in prison, on probation, or on parole (about 1.7 million) than were held as slaves in 1850 (870,000 or so). And with many more people of color than Whites being made felons by the criminal justice system, racial discrimination remains as common now as it was under slavery.

Social activist Angela Davis observes that the prison system is little more than a means for hiding society's ills. "Homelessness, unemployment, drug addiction, mental illness, and illiteracy are only a few of the problems that disappear from public view when the human beings contending with them are relegated to cages," she writes. "But prisons do not disappear problems, they disappear human beings. And the practice of disappearing vast numbers of people from poor, immigrant, and racially marginalized communities has literally become big business."

Because prison labor is the one exception to the Thirteenth Amendment codifying the abolition of slavery in the United States, in the wake of the Civil War, society simply substituted one form of involuntary servitude for another. With convicts required to work in just about every industry imaginable—agriculture, construction, manufacturing, bridge building, mining, and, of course, making license plates—punishment became profitable. Some inmates are even forced to work in slaughterhouses, perpetuating state-sanctioned violence while they serve time (and often suffering the same traumatic consequences as those paid to kill animals). Healthy prisoners who refuse to work face solitary confinement, loss of earned good time, and revocation of family visitation.

## From Schoolhouse to Jailhouse

The culture of discipline and punishment has become so normalized that it has even infiltrated our education system and developed into what has become known as the school-to-prison pipeline: the practice of pushing young students out of classrooms and into the juvenile and criminal justice systems. Schools criminalize the smallest infractions, such as not obeying a teacher's order, or profile certain students as "problem" youths. It's a pattern that results in the suspensions, expulsions, and arrests of millions of kids every year. In Arlington, Virginia, for example, two 10-year-old boys were suspended for three days for putting soapy water in their teacher's drink; felony charges carrying 20-year sentences were filed against them, though cooler heads prevailed and the charges were dropped.

Many urban and some suburban schools now approximate the prison experience, with a police or security presence, surveillance cameras, physical searches, and isolation from the larger community. An emphasis on zero-tolerance policies and control has replaced what was once an emphasis on learning and development. In such an environment, education's great democratizing effect—giving everyone the opportunity for upward mobility—is lost. Some students may be doomed before they've even learned their ABCs.

The pipeline is especially hard on students of color, those who identify as LGBTQ (Lesbian, Gay, Bisexual, Transgender, or Questioning), and those with disabilities. According to the US

Department of Education Office for Civil Rights, Black students are three times more likely to be expelled or suspended than White students, and students with disabilities are twice as likely to be suspended than their peers without disabilities.

Meanwhile, LGBTQ youth represent just 5 to 7 percent of the nation's overall youth population, but approximately 13 to 15 percent of those in the juvenile justice system self-identify as LGBTQ. These students may be three times more likely to experience criminal justice and school sanctions than youth who do not identify as LGBTQ. Once suspended from school, there is an increased likelihood that students will drop out entirely or commit crimes in their neighborhoods, leading to court involvement.

## Human Trafficking

The practice of trafficking people shares many similarities with animal exploitation, such as using violence or threats of violence to coerce compliance out of an unwilling victim (who may have been transported a long distance) to serve at the pleasure of humans. In the case of human trafficking, the "pleasure" derived is generally labor or sex. Forced labor may involve toiling on a farm or fishing boat, as we've seen, or in domestic servitude, health and beauty services, the production of illegal drugs, and other industries. In India, children as young as four years old smash coal in factories that churn out bricks for the nation's growing construction trade. They are there to pay off debts their elders incurred.

Often such "debts" are payments to the traffickers themselves, who bring workers into countries like the United States with promises of good wages, housing, and other benefits. According to the Urban Institute, labor-trafficking victims pay a "recruitment" fee averaging US$6150, which is more than the annual per-capita income in many of the nations they come from. Once in the US, workers are subjected to physical, mental, and/or financial abuse. A variety of "fees" are typically levied and deducted from paychecks, for instance, leaving workers without the means to pay back the initial amount "owed" to employers and recruiters for bringing them into the country. Consequently, victims are forced to remain enslaved.

Deceitful recruitment methods are also used to traffic victims into the sex trade. Women are enticed with offers of legitimate work—as a food server, perhaps, or a shop assistant or in the housekeeping department of a fancy hotel. Some are sold into trafficking by boyfriends, neighbors, or even relatives. Still others are promised marriage, an education, or other trappings of a better life somewhere. Once ensnared, a woman may be passed from one trafficker to another and moved further from her own country. Her passport or other documents are taken away, making her feel dependent upon her captors. Before she has been forced to "service" a client, the victim is often raped by the trafficker, beginning the cycle of physical abuse that commonly includes death threats, drugs, and physical and psychological torture. Traffickers even threaten the lives of the victims' families.

One reason that this type of slavery continues to flourish is that women and girls are seen as having little or no power, and it's in societies where women and girls are considered worthless that they are exposed to the greatest risk.

In addition to women and girls smuggled from other countries, pimps prey on runaways, foster children, and victims of physical and sexual abuse—anyone with vulnerabilities the pimp can use to control them. Women are commonly held against their wills in brothels or other rooms from which they cannot escape sexual servitude. Those who resist or don't "follow the rules" might be severely beaten or killed.

Often overlooked in the struggle against sex trafficking are the male victims—men and boys who comprise a relatively small but especially taboo segment of human slavery. Many studies estimate that women and girls account for 98 percent of those trafficked for forced commercial sexual exploitation worldwide, and men and boys make up 2 percent. But at least one study, released in 2008, suggests that boys could actually represent as much as 50 percent of the population of sex-trafficked children in the US.

Traffickers target marginalized populations—especially the homeless—and among the most vulnerable are LGBTQ youth, who are more likely to be kicked out of their homes because of their sexual orientation or gender identity. While 5 to 7 percent of the general youth population in the US self-identify as LGBTQ, they represent about 40 percent of homeless youth, making them statistically more likely to become victims of sex trafficking. A variety of factors can lead to being homeless, of course, but some 26 percent of homeless LGBTQ youth have been kicked out of their homes because their families rejected them for being LGBTQ-identified.

According to statistics gathered by Thorn, an agency that studies technology's role in sex trafficking, many young victims are bought and sold on some of the same sites consumers use to find a roommate, buy a used car, or look for a neighborhood garage sale. Thorn found that 70 percent of these children said they'd been advertised on websites such as Craigslist, where the trafficker posted a photo of the victim, some descriptive text, and a price.

## Capital Punishment

Among many social justice activists, the death penalty represents the ultimate human rights violation. It's also among the most controversial. While the immorality of such human rights abuses as genocide and slavery is generally beyond debate, capital punishment is even used by governments that claim to uphold principles of justice and equality. Citizens of the United States might criticize the hard-line rule of North Korea or Iran, yet they have to confront the reality that, like these countries, the US condemns people to death and carries out those judgments on a regular basis, as do China, Iraq, Yemen, Saudi Arabia, and scores of others. Indeed, China executes so many people that it stopped releasing its data in 2009, saying the number killed is a state secret. (Amnesty International estimates the nation puts thousands of people to death each year.)

Although many governments now reserve this punishment for those who commit murder, in some countries one can also be executed for homosexuality, adultery, renouncing one's faith, or practicing witchcraft. Methods of execution—which include hanging, lethal injection, gas chamber, electrocution, decapitation, firing squad, and stoning—vary from country to country and state to state, but all inflict emotional and physical suffering. Lethal injection, for instance, the execution method favored by most US states and the federal government, is far from being quick and painless. Indeed, it's become notorious for causing condemned prisoners to writhe in blistering pain for up to two hours. The last words of a man being put to death by injection in Oklahoma in 2014 were, "I feel my whole body burning."

Suffering is meted out long before the condemned reaches the gallows. Prisoners routinely spend decades awaiting execution on "death row" in conditions that amount to torture under international law: sensory deprivation, no contact with family, and held in solitary confinement.

Moreover, the death penalty is undeniably skewed to favor Whites and punish Blacks and Latinos. Of the 35 prisoners the US executed in 2014, two-thirds were people of color—17 Black men, five Latinos, and one Black woman. In one of many studies suggesting that the criminal justice system places more value on White lives than Black lives, researchers from Ohio State University found that Blacks convicted of killing Whites are not only more likely than White defendants to receive a death sentence, they are also more than twice as likely to be executed. Latinos, meanwhile, are 1.4 times more likely to be executed if they kill a White person.

In a truly sobering analysis covering the years 1976 to 2015, researchers in Louisiana concluded that Black men and boys comprise 61 percent of murder victims in the state, yet their killers have been executed in only three cases out of 12,949 homicides. Clearly, killing a White person is practically the only reason someone is executed there. (That the state's motto is "Union, Justice, and Confidence" is as ironic as it is insulting.)

The United States has a long history of expressing racial bias through the killing of Black men, women, and children. Among the first capital offenses codified in the eighteenth century that had not been borrowed from England were those made in response to the slave revolt of 1712: attempted murder and attempted rape committed by slaves became punishable by death.

Well into the twentieth century, the death penalty was being used for racial control. The case of George Stinney, a 14-year-old Black youth, remains one of the most haunting examples. Accused of killing two pre-teen White girls in March 1944, George was questioned without the presence of his parents or a lawyer and allegedly confessed to the murders. The boy maintained he was innocent, and his sister said they were together watching their family's cow graze near their house when the murders occurred. Regardless, after a two-hour trial, an all-White jury took just ten minutes to convict him, and he was sent to die in South Carolina's electric chair less than two months later. In 2014, a judge exonerated George Stinney, calling the trial and execution "a truly unfortunate episode in our history."

For lack of a better word, what happened to young George was a lynching, a form of racially motivated capital punishment that swept the South after the Civil War in an effort to preserve White supremacy. Following the passage of the Thirteenth Amendment in 1865, the US justice system held all races to be equal (at least in theory, if not in practice), meaning that Black defendants could no longer be put to death for such crimes as robbery, rape, or destroying property. Looking for a new way to oppress a population that was now considered free, White lynch mobs targeted Blacks for a host of perceived offenses, including business competition, vagrancy, and attempting to vote. Hanging, shooting, burning, or beating victims to death—all methods of "lynching"—became true acts of terrorism. By one estimate, between 1877 and 1950, 3959 Black men, women, and children were lynched in 12 Southern states. If we regard "lynchings" as extrajudicial punishments, they are clearly being used today by law enforcement, as we'll explore in Chapter 5.

Although capital punishment is touted as a way to curb crime, many studies show it does not have any impact on crime rates; indeed, we could reasonably argue that the death penalty is simply used as revenge. "One argument for the death penalty is that it is a strong deterrent to murder and other violent crimes. In fact, evidence shows just the opposite," wrote former US President Jimmy Carter in 2012. "The homicide rate is at least five times greater in the United States than in any Western European country, all without the death penalty... Southern states carry out more than 80 percent of the executions but have a higher murder rate than any other region. Texas has by far the most executions, but its homicide rate is twice that of Wisconsin, the first state to abolish the death penalty."

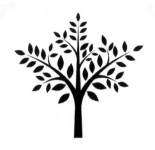

## Chapter 4

# On the Environment

*The generation that destroys the environment is not the generation that pays the price. That is the problem.*
—Wangari Maathai

There is arguably no tableau more emblematic of climate change and its impact on animals and the planet than that of a lone polar bear precariously perched on a melting ice floe. Such images— used by environmental groups to solicit donations and shared on social media sites to elicit outrage—have become increasingly common. Somewhere in a remote northern latitude, nature and humanity's habits converge in a dramatic Arctic scene that has become for many people proof positive that we've doomed our planet to ecological disaster as, one by one, plant and animal species disappear forever.

Actually, it's worse than one by one: the UN Environment Programme estimates that as many as 200 species of insect, bird, mammal, and plant become extinct *every day*. We are in the midst of the worst die-off since the dinosaurs suddenly vanished 65 million years ago, and unlike previous mass extinctions that were linked to natural events like evolutionary advances, climate shifts, volcanic eruptions, and asteroid strikes, *we* are to blame for the catastrophe that's happening even as you read this. The situation is so critical now that 99 percent of threatened species are at risk because of human activities such as habitat destruction, overpopulation, and hunting.

Two other major causes of species extinction, however—pollution and climate change—are driven largely by factory farming. From spewing ammonia, hydrogen sulfide, and methane into the air to creating massive manure lagoons that contaminate the water and soil, industrialized animal agriculture is responsible for much of the environmental degradation we have today. The role of meat, egg, and dairy foods in climate change has been quantified by a team of British researchers, who measured the amount of greenhouse gas (GHG) emissions created by various diets and concluded that omnivores are responsible for nearly 2.5 times as much global warming as vegans. Animal ag is not just a destroyer of species, but a chief reason our children and grandchildren will be inheriting a world with higher temperatures, shifting ocean currents, more frequent and destructive wildfires, rising seas, stronger storms, and more severe droughts.

## Animal Products and Climate Change

So, would going vegan solve climate change? The United Nations seems to think so. Ever since the UN released its 2006 report *Livestock's Long Shadow: Environmental Issues and Options*, in which the UN identified the production of animal-based foods as being responsible for 18 percent of GHG emissions—more than all of the carbon dioxide spewed by automobiles, boats, planes, and trains in the world combined—linking the meat and dairy industries to global warming and climate change has been a favorite way to denounce an omnivorous diet. According to the study, GHG emissions from animal agriculture are in the form of methane, which has 86 times more climate change potential than carbon dioxide, and nitrous oxide, which has 268 times more climate change potential. You can see how these stats could really add up.

Then a 2009 report from the Worldwatch Institute, *Livestock and Climate Change*, declared that when the entire life cycle and supply chain of the industry is taken into consideration, the annual GHG emissions that animal agriculture is responsible for actually amount to 51 percent. This report's authors recommend people consume plant-based foods instead of meat, eggs, and dairy products.

In 2015, the UN released another report, *Assessing the Environmental Impacts of Consumption and Production*, in which they urge "a substantial worldwide diet change, away from animal products" as a way to help curb climate change.

As with world hunger, the solution to climate change is more nuanced than meets the eye. But while experts quibble about just how much impact a vegan diet can have on the environment, common sense would seem to tell us that doing something that reduces cruelty while also helping to save the world from the worst impacts of climate change is an obvious step to take. As a bonus, an elimination of animals raised for food would also mitigate antibiotic-resistant infections, since about 80 percent of all antibiotics are currently used on farmed animals, and antibiotic-resistant bacteria can jump from animals to humans.

### Meat-Eating and Environmentalism

Many advocates in the vegan/animal rights movement consider how animal agriculture is slowly destroying ecosystems, not to mention the ozone layer. They will point out that consuming animals is environmentally unsustainable. They will cite how wasteful it is to produce food for animals and then eat the animals. They will argue that factory farms pollute the planet and use an extraordinary amount of water. And they conclude that no one who eats animals should call themselves an environmentalist.

On the face of it, such a conclusion seems sound. But let's not overlook some important points. For one thing, not every "meat eater" consumes the same amount of animal products. More and more people are adopting "veganish" diets that drastically reduce meat, eggs, and dairy foods. Yet these people would still be considered meat-eaters. Likewise, we need to remember that not all animal products put the same level of demand on resources. The environmental burden of producing meat from cows, for example, is significantly greater than producing meat from chickens. (And let's not forget: growing, harvesting, and transporting fruits and vegetables use vast resources, too.)

While I absolutely agree that eating lower on the food chain is better for the planet, how can we possibly know how the carbon footprint of a self-identified environmentalist measures up against that of a vegan? Consider the meat-eating environmentalist who commutes on a bike, carries her water in a reusable stainless-steel canteen, and whose meat habit consists of a cheeseburger once a month, versus a hardcore vegan who drives a gas-guzzling SUV, flies across the country multiple times a year, and whose hydration of choice comes in a never-ending series of disposable plastic bottles. Which of them probably has the lighter environmental impact?

I think it's important that we consider the consequences of criticizing another group for an apparent deficiency. Do we really believe we're building solidarity with the environmental movement when we try to shame them for what we perceive to be a shortcoming?

### Drought

Even as raising animals for food contributes to drought conditions, the industry makes matters worse by draining precious water supplies for hydrating, feeding, cleaning, and eventually slaughtering farmed animals. Let's take California as an example. My home state is no stranger to arid conditions (as I write this, we are in our fourth year of a severe drought), and we're the number-one dairy producer in the US with cows eating a substantial amount of alfalfa, which is an extremely water-intensive crop. By some estimates, nearly half the water in California's reservoirs and aquifers goes to animal agriculture. In addition to feeding West Coast bovines, farmers here are making hay by exporting alfalfa to China for that country's burgeoning dairy industry—and using some 100 billion gallons of water a year from the Colorado River to do so. That's enough water to supply the annual household needs of 1 million families.

In other words, industrialized animal agriculture helps create climate change, which in turn exacerbates drought, and then the companies take what little water is left to keep the ecologically destructive process going.

Although Big Ag is by far the biggest water guzzler, mainstream media tends to demonize other consumers when discussing drought, such as almond and orange growers. These crops, and many others, do use a substantial amount of water, but they are much more efficient than animal-based foods and thus kinder to the planet. It takes 106 gallons of water to produce just one ounce of beef, for example, while an ounce of almonds requires 23 gallons. Yes, that's a lot for a handful of nuts, but it's much better—and more compassionate—than what goes into raising and killing animals.

The crisis in California has gotten so bad that more than a dozen coastal cities are considering desalination plants, which make saltwater drinkable. It's an incredibly expensive option, and not without a host of other environmental concerns, such as the enormous carbon footprint each plant has and how they potentially harm marine life while sucking in millions of gallons of seawater each day. The drought issue alone should be enough to make a vegan of just about anyone who cares about the future of Earth.

## Wildlife on the Edge

When we consider how meat-eating impacts animals, we

naturally think of cows, chickens, pigs, and fishes, since these are among the many animals people consume. But wild (sometimes called "free-living") species are also affected, along with the environment they call home. In the Global North, this may be most evident in the United States, where beef barons have bullied their way into claiming more and more grazing land for cows — land also historically occupied by burros, horses, coyotes, and wolves. Those last two are apex predators, and it's not hyperbole to say ranchers hate them. Yes, ranchers hate burros and horses, too, but for a different reason: equines, they claim, compete with cows for forage and water. But the meat industry hates coyotes and wolves because these native carnivores literally eat ranchers' profits. Ironically, it was the ranchers and farmers who systematically killed antelope and buffalo — natural prey for wolves and coyotes — and replaced them with domesticated farmed animals. A hungry *Canis* doesn't much care if his meal was intended for human consumption or not.

For centuries now, ranchers have waged a violent though little-seen war against wild animals on rangeland, often with the help of the federal government. The USDA's oddly named Wildlife Services agency (which does nothing to serve wildlife) and the Bureau of Land Management (BLM) are the meat industry's hired guns — and taxpayers foot the bill. While Wildlife Services hunts down wolves and coyotes, often shooting these animals from helicopters, the BLM "manages" wild horse and burro populations by rounding up hundreds at a time, tearing apart equine families and social systems in the process. The fortunate ones are relocated to pastures or adopted out; others end up slaughtered to become food for a zoo's big cats or quietly shipped to Canada or Mexico, where the law allows horses to be killed for human consumption.

Wildlife Services, meanwhile, kills not only predators who threaten grazing cows, but species such as elk and deer to reserve more feed for cows. In addition to aerial gunning, the agency uses leghold traps, neck snares, and M-44s, devices that spew a cloud of sodium cyanide into the victim's mouth and nose, causing horrific suffering and sending toxic chemicals into the environment. Wildlife Services routinely ends up killing federally protected animals such as bald eagles, as well as dogs and cats, all of whom are considered collateral damage. They use explosives to destroy important habitat-creating animals like beaver, whose dams flood grazing land, often blowing up fishes and river otters as well.

But to the meat industry, wolves are the real "pest," and they vigorously defend their right to kill them to protect their interests. Whether ranchers genuinely believe killing these animals will prevent predation is anyone's guess, but a 2014 study examining 25 years of data found that using deadly force against wolves actually *increased* the chances of a wolf attacking cows by 5 to 6 percent, probably because killing a wolf disrupts the pack's behavior and prompts lone wolves to hunt beyond their territories. Sadly, the meat industry probably won't be happy until wolves and other animals who kill cows and sheep vanish from view. Indeed, such was the fate of the California grizzly bear, driven to extinction in the 1920s by hunters assisting ranchers and farmers.

Even when it doesn't intend to, the meat industry spawns environmental chaos, and it's been that way from the very beginning. Bringing heavy, hooved animals like bovines from Europe to graze in North America created an ecological nightmare. Unlike native mammals such as elk and deer who browse for their nourishment, cows tend to concentrate their grazing on one area, where they munch until there's nothing edible left. In the process, they trample vegetation along riverbanks, uproot native grasses and wildflowers and replace them with invasive weeds, destroy watersheds, and leave topsoils vulnerable to wind and water erosion. According to the Center for Biological Diversity, "In the arid Southwest, livestock grazing is the most widespread cause of species endangerment. By destroying vegetation, damaging wildlife habitats, and disrupting natural processes, livestock grazing wreaks ecological havoc on riparian areas, rivers, deserts, grasslands, and forests alike—causing significant harm to species and the ecosystems on which they depend."

Elsewhere, humanity's hunger for meat is wiping out entire species of flora and fauna as biodiverse countries—including those in Africa, Asia, and South America—clear more land to raise cows, goats, and sheep, and crops to feed these animals. The outlook is particularly bleak in tropical nations, home to the most biologically diverse ecosystems. Scientists estimate that if meat production continues to grow at its current rate, some countries may be using up to 50 percent more land as they attempt to satisfy demand, making meat the leading cause of species extinction, especially when combined with other impacts of the industry, such as climate change and pollution.

## Environmental Racism

Where concerns about the environment intersect with issues involving race, we're generally looking at environmental racism, a form of discrimination in which environmental hazards such as polluted air and contaminated drinking water disproportionately affect people of color, who may also lack access to healthcare. Farm workers and their children, for instance, are routinely doused with pesticides sprayed onto nearby crops, while families living or working close to factory farms commonly suffer respiratory problems, headaches, fly infestations in their homes, and increased incidents of depression and fatigue from the toxic stew that animal agriculture generates every day. It's particularly bad in the eastern half of North Carolina, where thousands of industrial pig farms—each with a massive, open cesspool to collect manure—are clustered in Black, Latino, and Native American communities and subject them to a barrage of health problems, fouled water, and feces spewed onto laundry left outside to dry.

And it's not just industrialized farms creating a problem. Because segregation continues to divide many communities along racial lines, non-White residents are most often those who live where polluting developments such as municipal landfills, rail stations, junkyards, congested highways, garbage dumps, and coal plants are sited. In addition, these neighborhoods may be characterized by high poverty, deteriorating infrastructure, dilapidated housing, urban decay, inadequate schools, and chronic unemployment.

Some critics of the environmental justice movement have rejected the assertion that these conditions have anything to do with racism, yet a 2014 study shows that, in fact, they do. Researchers from the University of Minnesota investigated environmental injustice and inequality in residential outdoor nitrogen dioxide ($NO_2$) air pollution for the contiguous US population and found that people of color breathe 38 percent more $NO_2$ than do White people. $NO_2$ is emitted mainly from combustion in vehicles and power plants and causes heart conditions as well as asthma and other respiratory diseases. The study's authors estimate the disparity in exposure is equal to some 7000 deaths a year from heart disease, and it is even greater than the inequality for income. Nationwide, people of color are more exposed than Whites in even the cleanest cities, the study says, though as the size and population density of a metropolitan area grows, race becomes an even bigger factor. Clearly, it's not just the difference between lower- and higher-income levels; the results suggest that even wealthy people of color tend to reside in communities that are environmentally worse off than neighborhoods occupied by impoverished White people.

As a leading campaigner against environment racism, Robert D. Bullard observes that eight out of every ten African Americans live in neighborhoods where they are in the majority. "Residential segregation decreases for most racial and ethnic groups with additional education, income and occupational status," he says. "However, this scenario does not hold true for African Americans. African Americans, no matter what their educational or occupational achievement or income level, are exposed to higher crime rates, less effective educational systems, high mortality risks, more dilapidated surroundings and greater environmental threats because of their race. For example, in the heavily populated South Coast air basin of the Los Angeles area, it is estimated that over 71 percent of African Americans and 50 percent of Latinos reside in areas with the most polluted air, while only 34 per cent of whites live in highly polluted areas."

When it comes to examples of areas where people of color are environmentally impacted, it would be difficult to find a more catastrophic location than the Gulf Coast of the United States, where in August of 2005 Hurricane Katrina killed 1836 people—most of them Black—and displaced tens of thousands more, along with their companion animals. The biggest loss of life occurred in New Orleans after the storm passed and the city's poorly engineered levee system failed, sending a massive surge of water into flood-prone neighborhoods. Most of the areas that were completely washed out were lower-elevation communities of working-class poor and districts populated by Black educated professionals and business owners. Meanwhile, areas of higher elevation, such as the French Quarter, Uptown, and the Garden District—and populated primarily by White residents—were spared the worst of Katrina. These neighborhoods offered residents convenient access to public transportation and adequate urban infrastructure and generally did not force them to accept environmental burdens, such as the overhead highways or industrial canals common in the poorer parts of the city.

I think it's safe to say that for most Black people in the United States, a polar bear on a melting ice floe is not the face of climate change—it's Katrina. Scientists and environmental activists tell us that warming oceans are going to intensify storms like the one that hit New Orleans, and those who are economically, socially, politically, culturally, institutionally, or otherwise marginalized will be the most vulnerable. The tragic irony is that it's often in the very communities where they live that we find the toxic facilities fueling this devastation.

"Hurricane Katrina and its aftermath taught us that the coming ecological disasters will hit the poor first and worst. More of us are beginning to see that there can be no separation between our concern for vulnerable people and our concern for a vulnerable planet," says environmental advocate Van Jones, who adds that Blacks, Latinos, and Asians should be deeply invested in the health of the planet. "To put it bluntly," he says, "people of color have much more directly at stake in the greening of America than white college students do." And as for imperiled Arctic megafauna, Jones says, "This country can save the polar bears and poor kids too."

Environmental racism is not limited to the United States, of course. The globalization of the world's economy has led to the degradation of habitats and living areas for human populations around the planet. But as with the US, it is the Indigenous peoples and other people of color living downstream and downwind from what the privileged can afford to avoid who are hit the hardest. Forest destruction for a product such as palm oil, for example, ultimately deprives local communities of their right to a healthy environment. By systematically eliminating the natural resources Indigenous peoples rely on, palm oil companies often create food insecurity and rob the region's human inhabitants of their livelihoods. Moreover, the industry's liberal use of toxic fertilizers and chemicals—including some 25 different pesticides, herbicides, and insecticides—contaminates the soil, groundwater, and crops, while tons of untreated palm oil-mill effluent is discharged into rivers and seeps into the terrain. And as fires flatten the timbered landscape to make way for meticulous rows of oil palm trees, the region is shrouded in a smoky fog, forcing people to wear masks.

Although much of the environmental destruction seen in the world is due to food production, such as the enormous growth of factory farms and clear-cutting land to grow oil palm trees or feed for farmed animals, other industries contribute to the devastation. The manufacture of chemicals, mining for minerals and natural resources, timber extraction, and power plants all create toxic environments, pollute groundwater, and contaminate soil, turning villages and towns throughout the world into toxic communities. Making matters worse, many of these polluting industries are owned and operated by international corporations, which enjoy tax breaks, influence in local government, and the use of valuable land and water supplies, among other special benefits.

## Ecofeminism

In exploring a vegan ethic and its relationship to the environment, we should consider not only how animal agriculture impacts climate change, disrupts ecological harmony, and destroys ecosystems, but how humanity's dominance and perceived superiority over the natural world prevents us from seeing the intrinsic value of nature. Ecofeminists understand this, and it's here that we find a lens through which we can view environmental and gender issues side by side. Although we looked at ecofeminism a bit in the previous chapter, I would be remiss not to include this philosophy in our discussion here.

As the name implies, ecofeminism links ecological and feminist concerns: ecofeminists see the natural world as a feminist issue and in turn address feminist issues in relation to Earth. An activist and academic movement, ecofeminism recognizes that the exploitation and oppression of nature is fundamentally connected to the exploitation and oppression of women, people of color, and other non-dominant groups. Consequently, efforts to help the environment should overlap with work to overcome the oppression of humans.

One way they approach this link is to expose the patriarchal dualisms that separate the world into opposing pairs of concepts, where the first concept is thought of as superior, and the other, inferior one is discriminated against: masculine/feminine, White/Black, mind/body, reason/emotion, human/nonhuman, culture/nature, civilized/primitive, etc. Through such thinking— which some ecofeminists also refer to as the "logic of domination"—nature is considered something to be "mastered by men," especially White men, who also seek to objectify and dominate women, people of color, and animals. Thus, we find this "good/bad" logic used to support systems of oppression beyond the exploitation of the environment, including sexism, racism, and speciesism. Just as they control female bodies (human and nonhuman) for their own gains, patriarchy feminizes the natural world ("Mother Nature," "Mother Earth," "fertile soil," etc.) and turns it into an economic resource to be consumed.

Ecofeminism, then, seeks to dismantle these dualisms and think critically about humanity's role in the systematic subordination of other humans and the environment. It wasn't until I met Marti Kheel, co-founder of Feminists for Animal Rights, that I really appreciated the concept of ecofeminism. Marti, who left the world in 2011, had a beautiful home in the Bay Area, and she hosted a number of brainstorming sessions in her living room to help her friend, the prolific author Jeffrey Masson, hash out thoughts for his books dealing with veganism. I was fortunate to participate in two of these sessions, and each time the room was filled with some of the most renowned names in the movement. What I remember most, though, was how Marti, with her quiet warmth, would welcome everyone and keep the conversation flowing. She also had one of the most extensive private animal rights libraries I have ever seen, and lauren and I are proud to have several of these books with us now.

But it was Marti's own writing that inspired my interest in ecofeminism, in particular her 2008 book *Nature Ethics: An Ecofeminist Perspective*, in which she observed that certain (male) nature ethicists have stressed the importance of seeing human beings as different from nature. But achieving this means we alienate ourselves from the natural world when in reality we yearn to connect with it. The result, explained Marti, is an urge to satisfy that desire through control and violence, such as hunting animals in the wild. (That same impulse to conquer nature is evident in circuses and marine parks, where humans "train" animals to perform stunts they'd never do except under the threat of violence or having their food withheld.)

Environmental justice and feminism also intersect within issues involving women's health. When fast-food chain KFC teamed with a well-known breast cancer nonprofit organization to sell buckets of chicken legs, breasts, and other body parts, for example, ecofeminists called it a clear case of pinkwashing—a term coined by the group Breast Cancer Action—which is applying the breast cancer symbol (a pink ribbon) onto products to generate sales to consumers who believe their purchase will fight the deadly disease. Not only was the partnership criticized for encouraging purchases of a product that can be linked to breast cancer, but KFC locates its stores in low-income communities that disproportionately suffer from health issues such as diabetes, obesity, and cancer. A similar pinkwashing campaign featured Yoplait yogurt, which at the time was manufacturing its products using milk from cows who were given rBGH, a bovine growth hormone associated with an increased risk of breast cancer.

## Healthy You, Healthy Planet

There are plenty of reasons to embrace a vegan ethic, and certainly love of our environment is among them. As individual parts of a larger whole, we have a responsibility not only to ourselves but also to those with whom we share the planet—and indeed to the planet itself. While the health benefits of a plant-based diet have long been recognized, it's only recently that its environmental impact has been established. A 571-page scientific report from the USDA's Dietary Guidelines Advisory Committee published in 2015, for example, specifically states that an organic vegan diet has the lowest impact on resources and ecosystem quality.

From the use of water to produce food to the vast amount of waste and pollution animal agriculture generates, veganism is clearly better for everyone. Here are some additional realities to consider:

- It takes 450 gallons of water to produce a hamburger versus 13 gallons to grow an orange.
- One gallon of cow's milk requires 880 gallons of water.
- Farmed animals account for at least 32,000 million tons of carbon dioxide per year—51 percent of all worldwide greenhouse gas emissions.
- Farmed animals are responsible for 65 percent of all emissions of nitrous oxide, a greenhouse gas 296 times more destructive than carbon dioxide that stays in the atmosphere for 150 years.
- Each lactating cow used in the dairy industry produces about 150 pounds of manure a day, thus generating 330 pounds of nitrogen, 56 pounds of phosphorus, and 36 pounds of potassium. Despite this, factory farms have largely escaped pollution regulations.
- A person exchanging a meat-eating diet for a vegan diet reduces his or her carbon emissions by 1.5 metric tons a year.
- Every second, 1.5 acres of rainforest are cleared.
- Farmed animals and crops grown to feed them are the leading causes of rainforest destruction.

Thus far we've looked at animal rights, veganism, human rights, and the environment and how they coincide. But it's one thing to frame these movements as sharing commonalities with other spheres of oppression. It's more challenging—and indeed more critical—to explore how these entanglements might be used to build coalitions and make strides toward abolishing oppressive institutions worldwide. Think of the following chapter, then, as a roadmap to a future in which a vegan ethic becomes not an abstract ideal, but a mechanism for achieving the world of peace, justice, and equality we've been struggling for.

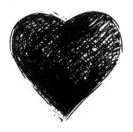

**Chapter 5**

# On a More Compassionate World

*Until we have the courage to recognize cruelty for what it is—whether its victim is human or animal—we cannot expect things to be much better in this world.*
—Rachel Carson

For me and many others, the essence of a vegan ethic is compassion. Putting that into practice can mean expanding your definition of "cruelty free," recognizing how your privileges as a consumer can effect change, and then acting accordingly. As the Buddhist monk and peace activist (and vegan) Thich Nhat Hanh has said, "Compassion is a verb."

I believe that to ignore the rights of humans and other animals—that is, denying them their dignity and liberty or otherwise abusing them—is to dismiss how we are all in need of liberation. The unity of suffering connects species, races, genders, classes, and religions in a very tangible way. They do not exist in a vacuum. We will not rid ourselves of one type of oppression while allowing another to flourish. It simply cannot happen.

Yet the position of some human rights activists who agree with the animal rights cause is that they are too busy to devote time to advocating on behalf of nonhumans. But helping animals need not require any additional time. By going vegan—eating plant-based foods, wearing clothing not made from animals, avoiding products tested on animals, and not patronizing businesses that exploit *anyone*—you become an agent of change.

Likewise, vegans and animal activists can take a stand against the oppression of disenfranchised humans. We can begin by not using language that demonizes non-White cultures: Chinese people are "barbarians" because they eat dogs; Spaniards are "uncivilized" because they go to bullfights; Mexicans are "sadistic" for supporting *charreadas* (rodeos); Africans are "evil" because they kill elephants; and so on. Nowhere in these diatribes is there any mention that most of the citizens in a given country usually disagree with the cruelty—or that nations in the West are responsible for many more atrocities.

## Building Coalitions

But I think a vegan ethic calls upon us to do more than just check our language. As we've discussed, different oppressions go hand in hand (and paw and fin and claw), and only through solidarity and rejecting *all* discrimination will we achieve linked liberations. Such is the promise held by building coalitions among movements, each of which must recognize and advocate for the rights of those beyond the scope of its own unique mission. Coalition efforts are responsible for some of the world's most important—though imperfect—progressive reforms, including child labor laws enacted after the mobilization efforts of unions, religious groups, and children's advocates, and the 1964 Civil Rights Act and 1965 Voting Rights Act, passed after labor activists joined forces with the civil rights movement.

The liberation movements, however, have yet to catch up. Animal rights groups should include as an active part of their agenda the struggle for gay rights, women's rights, or civil rights—or, better yet, all of them. Equally important, an organization working to dismantle human rights abuses ought to be fighting speciesism as well.

We are seeing some progress. In addition to Food Empowerment Project, which works to empower people through their myriad food choices, and Sistah Vegan Project, which focuses on how systems of oppression operate, there is VINE Sanctuary, an ecofeminist LGBTQ-run nonprofit that rescues chickens, cows, and other animals while working to facilitate alliances among animal, environmental, and social justice activists. Our Hen House is an animal rights nonprofit organization that also campaigns for gay and lesbian rights. A Well-Fed World's dual mission is to feed families while also advocating a plant-based diet. The group #Not1More challenges unjust immigration laws and gives a voice to day laborers, LGBTQ undocumented immigrants, and others impacted by deportation. Black Women For Wellness, meanwhile, focuses on reproductive, racial, gender, and environmental justices. And there are others that take a more inclusive approach to liberation.

Sadly, one reason these groups are so exceptional is that they are, well, the exception. The animal rights community is chiefly—though not exclusively—led and shaped by White men who are leading and shaping a movement predominately comprised of White females. The movement's women are all too often objectified in the name of fighting speciesism and are featured in sexist campaigns that rely on one type of oppression to raise awareness about another. Gendered hierarchies within the animal liberation movement are responsible for some of this, but not all.

A number of women (and some men) are changing the course of the movement, however. They recognize that a lot of animal rights activists disregard campaigns beyond animal liberation, believing their efforts should be focused exclusively on the plight of animals used for food, entertainment, research, etc. Our grandparents called this kind of myopic attitude "Not seeing the forest for the trees." Today we call it being "single issue," and every major movement has members who practice it. By single issue, I mean focusing on one problem to the exclusion—and often the expense—of others, failing to recognize how the problem fits into a larger context with intersecting issues and movements.

Being single issue is boycotting Canadian "seafood" until Canada stops killing seals.

Being single issue is using sexist imagery to promote an anti-bullfighting campaign.

Being single issue is buying a beverage because it's vegan, but giving no consideration to the unjust practices of the company that produced it, which may include mistreating workers, privatizing water, and polluting the environment.

Single-issue activism fails because focusing on one social justice issue ignores and marginalizes other people and groups, and it denies us a clearer perspective on injustices and how we can create solutions. It also robs us of important coalitions and solidarity with other movements. I am reminded of a story Joyce Tischler, founder of the Animal Legal Defense Fund, once told me. In 1981, Joyce learned that the US Navy had shot and killed more than 600 feral burros at its Weapons Testing Center in China Lake, California, and planned to kill 5000 more. Joyce wasn't even sure what a burro was, but she spent an entire night typing a series of pleadings arguing that, under the National Environmental Policy Act, the Navy could not kill the burros without preparing an environmental impact statement. It took eight months of work, but eventually she won the case. A little help from environmental groups would have been nice, Joyce said, but they considered the animals "pests" who were eating endangered desert plants.

I am not suggesting that focusing your efforts on a specific campaign within a specific movement is a bad idea—clearly that's what Joyce was doing for the burros. What I am saying is that being exclusive about any form of oppression—such as only regarding anti-speciesist campaigns as being worthwhile—

fosters the notion that what one group does is worse than what others do. Are Japan's citizens "monsters" because of the Taiji dolphin drives? Of course not. Many Japanese aren't even aware of these annual hunts, and many of those who are aware protest against them. So hate speech deriding "those people" as being heartless or greedy or fill-in-the-blank is at best intolerant and at worst racist.

Some organizations mobilizing for change believe that taking a position on a struggle outside their comfort zones—such as an environmental group helping an animal rights group or advocating a vegan diet—could alienate their supporters who might feel conflicted about the issue. Yet doesn't it seem probable that having a wider circle of compassion and considering a broader range of inequities would attract more members, even as some with a narrower view depart?

## Normalizing Speciesism

Among the themes of this book is that we can't consider any form of oppression in isolation because they are all connected by privilege, control, and economic power, often backed up by violence or the threat of violence. While there is no hierarchy of oppression—they are all reprehensible—as the late activist and author Norm Phelps observed, speciesism is the one form of oppression whose oppressors consist of members of every other oppressed, non-vegan group. Consequently, while other injustices serve to divide humanity into groups (privileged/ White/male/heterosexual versus marginalized/Black/female/ LGBTQ, for instance), speciesism unites people. Nonhuman animal exploitation offers a veritable smorgasbord of human "benefits"—food, clothing, entertainment, scientific research, you name it—and rare is the person who doesn't see these as enhancing the quality of her/his life. Eating and wearing animals are the reality for most people.

Indeed, systems of oppression are structured around what are understood to be societal "norms," and society considers few things to be more normal than using and consuming animals. As a result, the animal liberation message is often lost on other social justice activists, who may have difficulty identifying with nonhuman victims, especially when they perceive themselves as benefitting from them. Unlike other forms of oppression, animal abuse is one that "benefits" some 97 percent of the population. So in addition to overcoming the concerns of members of some devalued groups, including the feminist and Black communities, to whom even the word "animal" can have a negative connotation, anti-speciesism activists may struggle to find ways to create solidarity with other movements.

pattrice jones beautifully articulates this struggle in her 2014 book *The Oxen at the Intersection*, which examines how a number of diverse advocates converged in a campaign to save the lives of two oxen, Bill and Lou, who, yoked side by side, had tilled the farm at a small Vermont college for a decade. College officials considered the aging animals to be worthless and wanted to turn them into hamburgers. When news of these plans hit the media, pattrice tried to broker a compassionate solution by offering Bill and Lou retirement at VINE Sanctuary, but college officials were adamant that the oxen be "used for another purpose," which meant butchering them and serving their remains in the student dining hall.

Her narrative involves not only speciesism, but racism, sexism, homophobia, and even ableism: Lou had stepped into a gopher hole, suffered the bovine equivalent of a sprained ankle, and was destined for slaughter because the college no longer regarded him as "able-bodied." Implicit in our understanding of "rights" is that our capabilities confer basic rights on us, and if we fail to be "valuable" members of society—we commit a crime and go to prison, for example, or we become disabled—our rights can be taken away. We no longer possess moral standing. Such is the case with individuals like Lou who are denied basic rights (such as life, liberty, and control over their bodies) because they lack particular abilities and are thus victims of ableism. "It's not merely that the most common rationale used to justify human dominion over animals is *similar* to the rationale used to excuse the mistreatment of people with disabilities," writes pattrice. "It is the *exact same* argument!"

The ultimately unsuccessful efforts of everyone trying to rescue Bill and Lou (the college killed Lou in November 2012, and Bill mysteriously vanished from public view) now serve as a model of how activists can agitate from very different perspectives. *Oxen* may be an example of how *not* to engage in a campaign that involves so many angles—species, gender, race, male privilege, and class among them. Indeed, pattrice admits there are tactics she and other activists could have employed that might have resulted in a happy outcome. The lesson here is that by carefully analyzing a given situation and building coalitions, rather than relying on a one-size-fits-all strategy, we stand a better chance of success.

### *Fractured Front*

In attempting to build coalitions, it's critical that we are careful not to co-opt the message of another group or, worse, insult them. In 2012, for instance, a movement called Black Lives Matter was created to call attention to the anti-Black racism permeating the United States. It was prompted by the murder of Trayvon Martin, a Black teen who was shot as he was simply walking home one night and whose killer was acquitted, and it is intended to widen the conversation around state violence to include all of the ways in which Black people are intentionally left powerless. This tactic to (re)build the Black liberation movement has helped bring attention to the many Black men, women, and children who are extrajudicially killed by police or vigilante law enforcement—one every 28 hours in the US.

After the launch of Black Lives Matter, it didn't take long for the words "All Lives Matter" to appear on social media, and it's been used by the animal rights movement in an apparent attempt to be inclusive. Actually, they managed to both appropriate and negate Black Lives Matter at the same time. Perhaps the animal advocates misinterpreted the slogan to mean that Black people don't believe nonhuman animals matter. Or maybe they were trying to expand the message (as if racism is too narrow a topic). Whatever the intention, members of the African-American community rightly read "All Lives Matter" as "Black Lives *Don't* Matter."

This is hardly the only example of how the animal rights movement has tried to align itself with racism. In trying to compare the oppression of nonhuman animals with the oppression of Blacks, White people in the movement often argue that both are disfavored groups that have been enslaved and have suffered extreme discrimination. But as I've mentioned earlier, to a group that was held to not be human as a way for their oppressors to justify slavery—and who are still called "animals" and "beasts"—this comparison does not have the desired effect of elevating nonhumans, but serves to degrade and alienate Blacks. Likewise, however terribly animals have suffered in the meat industry, a gentile referring to their slaughter as a "Holocaust" or "genocide" does not endear the cause to the Jewish community, for whom any suggestion of Nazi death camps carries a lingering and unspeakable pain. Even if they bear similarities, agonies such as human slavery and the Jewish Holocaust should not be compared with the exploitation and killing of nonhuman animals. I believe this only serves to hold us back from crossing over into a mainstream movement.

## Cultivating Compassion

With its roots in Latin, the word *compassion* literally means "to suffer together." Those of us who are highly empathetic know this well, for we vicariously experience others' pain intensely. I cannot see animals lying on the side of the road, for example, without anguishing over their deaths and the loss their loved ones must feel. And watching documentaries about the civil rights movement fills me with the shame wrought by centuries of privileged White people subjecting Black people to the most shameful brand of exploitation and discrimination. I know I'm not alone. Research shows that ethical vegans and vegetarians respond with more empathy to the suffering of humans and other animals than omnivores do.

Many psychologists will tell you that having empathy isn't a choice—either someone has it or they don't. Some will go on to say that we as a society are becoming less empathetic. These critics explain that mobile devices have become a substitute for face-to-face interaction, gradually inclining us toward a social laziness in which we cease to be part of a real-life community and care for nothing but our own welfare. Because our brains evolved to consider the needs of the group, rather than just ourselves, they say, the isolation of staring at a digital screen is creating a culture of self-absorbed misfits.

While I can certainly see the value of spending quality time away from the Internet and mobile devices, I can't quite buy the theory that being online makes us less empathetic. Nor do I agree that empathy is a trait you're either born with or you're not. I think empathy is a choice, and there's a growing body of evidence to support my belief. According to these studies, any perceived "limits" to our compassion—such as having the time and ability to only care about nonhuman animals—can change, depending on what we *want* to feel.

We can, for example, decide to not feel empathy for a group of victims, as was illustrated by a study that measured a phenomenon known as the "collapse of compassion." Researchers wanted to understand why people will express outrage over the abuse of an individual, yet paradoxically display little or no sympathy for large-scale suffering (think humanitarian crisis or factory farming). Among their conclusions is that people restrain their responses (if subconsciously) when faced with tragedies they expect will overwhelm them emotionally. The more awareness people have of the processes they use to regulate their response to mass suffering, say the study's authors, the more control over them they are likely to have. In other words, we can learn to exhibit more empathy—a revelation that highlights the importance of children's natural love for animals and encouraging that compassion throughout their lives, rather than trying to stifle it once they learn where meat really comes from.

More evidence that empathy can be traced to nurture, not nature, comes from research in the United States indicating that the country has a serious empathy deficit problem, with levels of compassion toward others on the decline since the 1980s. Such a drop would indicate people are influencing their own empathy. This intrigued researchers at Stanford University, who looked at the issue in 2014. They found that when people discovered that empathy was an ability that could be enhanced, rather than a permanent personality trait, they exerted more effort to experience empathy for racial groups other than their own. And it worked.

### *An Exercise in Empathy*
Living fully—and helping others do the same—means acknowledging pain and inequity, whether we're outraged by the injustice of an animal in a cage, a woman victimized by prejudice, or a child forced into slavery. It's natural for us to feel compassion for these victims. But what about someone who might not seem to us to be a victim—someone who is an active participant in a cruelty we abhor? I'm going to ask you to consider doing something you probably don't believe you can—or at least don't want to: feel compassion for a slaughterhouse worker. Did I not concede earlier in this book that this is a challenging goal?

In Chapter 3 we looked at how those who are paid to kill animals might themselves be abused and oppressed. These are often undocumented workers who have been duped into coming to a new country with the promise of well-paid employment. What awaits them are institutionalized violence and dangerous, filthy working and living conditions that only the most financially desperate person would endure. It's the ultimate dead-end job without any hope of advancement. Many have little or no knowledge of the local language, so they usually don't understand their rights.

Industrial cogs performing their lethal business inside an invisible killing machine, slaughterhouse workers are kept hidden from the public. Until a video depicting them beating and mocking animals is recorded by an undercover activist and released to the media, that is. Then there is an immediate outcry from the community, from animal lovers, and even from the slaughterhouse management, who nearly always try to distance themselves from the taint of abuse by claiming their "humane" standards are the highest and blaming the crimes on a few "bad apples."

The cruelty I've seen in these kinds of videos is inexcusable, and it sickens me. But look, if you dare, at the faces of those men angrily abusing the animals. They are almost always the low-paid, immigrant workers. They take their cues from the bosses, and the bosses treat them with disdain. They are berated and exploited and threatened.

Such mistreatment is nothing new, and it was brought to the public's attention in 1906 with the publication of *The Jungle*, Upton Sinclair's groundbreaking exposé of the Chicago meatpacking trade. Within his stomach-turning narrative of unsanitary sausage production and heartbreaking animal deaths, Sinclair writes of a Lithuanian immigrant who is abused by his employer as he is paid a pittance to perform the most repulsive tasks in the slaughterhouse. (*The Jungle* eventually led to food safety legislation, though Sinclair's goal with the book was actually to raise awareness about how the workers were treated, not the animals. Today, the propensity for those who participate in or witness the routine slaughter of animals to commit violent crimes is known as the "Sinclair Effect.")

I am not suggesting that we ignore the cruelties these workers commit. But I think the animal rights movement targets them and celebrates their arrests because it's easy and it puts a face on abuse—faces that are often those of people of color. In considering the exploitation of these people alongside the animals they are exploiting, we glimpse not only the institutionalized hierarchy of domination, but the cycle of oppression, with the abuse of workers getting passed on to the abuse of animals. Slaughterhouse workers are another link in the food system's long chain of inhumane treatment.

By publicly naming and shaming these animal abusers, the animal liberation movement overlooks a tremendous opportunity to build alliances with other groups, including those that work with people of color, victims of domestic violence, and immigrant populations, to name but a few. If you still find it intolerable to feel any compassion for those whose livelihood depends on such an odious and reprehensible task, you may be interested to know that many former slaughterhouse workers have rejected their pasts and turned into vocal animal advocates, including Virgil Butler in the United States, Kim Stallwood in England, and Carl Scott in New Zealand.

## *Benefits of Compassion*

The practice of compassion is a gift to those (human or nonhuman) whose suffering you wish to relieve, of course, but it's also a gift to yourself. Compassion imbues our lives with meaning, and studies have shown that benevolence toward others increases our happiness and health and makes us less inclined to be fearful of life's pains. It also doubles your body's level of DHEA (the anti-aging hormone), while reducing cortisol (the stress hormone) by 23 percent. If you have a spiritual practice, you probably have already seen how compassion enhances that aspect of your life, as well.

All this means that compassionate people may experience greater psychological well-being while enjoying healthier, happier, more fulfilling, and even longer lives. For many people, giving to others is as pleasurable, if not more so, than receiving. And it stands to reason that expanding our circles of compassion will exponentially increase the numerous benefits acts of kindness bestow.

Other research indicates that it's not enough to simply do good — one must do so with the right intention. A study by Sara Konrath at the University of Michigan's Institute for Social Research revealed that while people who volunteer *do* have longer life spans than those who don't, the longevity is only the result of volunteering for altruistic, rather than self-serving, reasons. Researchers Barbara Fredrickson and Steve Cole and their colleagues demonstrated this outcome on a biological level. Their study found that people who have high levels of what is known as *eudaimonic* well-being, which comes from having a deep sense of purpose and meaning in life, had low levels of the cellular inflammation associated with many diseases, including cancer and heart disease. In contrast, they found that people who had high levels of *hedonic* well-being, which is happiness attained through instant gratification, had high levels of that unhealthy cellular inflammation.

## Making Excuses

In yet another study — one that helps explain why people eat meat — an international team of researchers found that omnivores use a variety of psychological mechanisms (let's call them what they are: excuses) to rationalize their consumption of animals. Among the excuses they use, four of them are so popular that the researchers labeled them "the 4Ns." Study participants either justified their meat-eating by saying that human bodies require it (the "Necessary" excuse, the most common), that humans are natural carnivores (the "Natural" excuse), that almost everyone does it (the "Normal" excuse), or that meat tastes good (the "Nice" excuse).

What does all this have to do with compassion? Well, the study also indicated that the more people believe in these excuses, the more likely they are to reject the suffering of others. Men in the study embraced the 4Ns more than women, which of course is consistent with what we know about the demographics of the animal liberation movement, and the more meat a person consumed, the more likely they were to use one of the 4Ns as an excuse.

Moreover, the study's authors found that meat-eaters were generally uncompromising in their rationalizations, which the authors explain can "lead people to overestimate the amount of evidence that favors their position." In other words, meat-eaters often force themselves to minimize the impact their diets can have on the world as a whole. The authors observe that many of humanity's worst cultural practices have endured because of the same rationalizations we create for eating animals.

Think of it this way: In the United States, it was once considered "Necessary" to deny women the right to vote, "Natural" to own another human being, "Normal" to prohibit same-sex and interracial marriages, and "Nice" to use heroin as an ingredient in children's cough syrup. The excuses for these practices seem ridiculous to us now. Well, to most of us. While many other appalling practices continue to flourish, it's clear that the excuses people use for them—like the commonalities of oppression inherent in their foundation—are connected. Moving past these excuses is essential to embracing a life of compassion.

## Beyond Excuses

There are myriad reasons why humans rationalize unhealthy and selfish behaviors. Clearly, many people suffer from cognitive dissonance when it comes to what they eat. People are also notoriously lazy; their behaviors become habits that are hard to break. We feel safe in our comfort zones and find it's easier to simply ignore the truth, reasoning that life is hard enough as it is. Why worry about a child being forced to harvest cocoa pods in Western Africa, for instance, when you've found a vegan chocolate you really like? I remember being at a restaurant with someone who ordered breaded chicken for dinner, and when I started to tell her how chickens are treated in the meat industry, she scowled and blurted, "Stop! I don't want to know!" For her, living in denial was easier than having to acknowledge her complicity in harming animals, whom she claimed to love. She, like so many other consumers, chose convenience over conscience.

Fear also plays a significant role in the excuses we make—fear of repercussions, fear of change, and especially fear of the unknown. A man might fear what his friends would think of him if he were to speak out on behalf of a female co-worker who's being sexually harassed, for example, so he tells himself it's none of his business. Someone with a bias against gays and lesbians might fear the social transformation of marriage equality. Or an omnivore might fear the unfamiliarity of a plant-based diet. (I don't mean to simplify any of these attitudes, just to illustrate how fear can be a factor that informs our choices.)

The first step to removing these obstacles to compassion is to recognize the excuses you are making. Each justification, defense, and rationalization you hold onto is a way to resist doing something that fear or habit tells you to avoid. It took me years to finally make the leap from vegetarian to ethical vegan because I enjoyed eggs and dairy foods. I told myself I was already saving the lives of hundreds of animals by not eating them and that I could never bake desserts or enjoy ice cream again if I were to go vegan.

Next, trust your authentic self. You are reading this book because you care, so it's clear you are open to learning and expanding your compassion. Allow yourself to be vulnerable and to make mistakes. It was when I lowered my barriers and did something I feared by visiting a sanctuary for farmed animals that I let go of my egg and dairy excuses. Yes, I was actually afraid to visit a sanctuary, because I suspected meeting hens and cows rescued from the egg and dairy industries would change me, and I wasn't ready for change; indeed, I was secretly hoping that someone at the sanctuary would assure me I was just fine the way I was and I could go on living and eating in my comfort zone. But that same voice that whispered to me in Pamplona a decade earlier was tugging at my sleeve again, nudging me to live up to a higher standard.

Step three is to find ways to make your choices deeply fulfilling; this will ensure you enjoy the benefits that come with rejecting excuses. In my case, not only did my sanctuary visit help me to stop making excuses and go vegan, but I discovered just how easy it is to bake without eggs and how delicious non-dairy ice creams are. Veganism has given me flavors and culinary experiences I never imagined, while making me feel better— emotionally, physically, and spiritually—than ever before.

Finally, be patient with yourself. Eliminating excuses in your life isn't going to happen overnight. But as you replace passive rationalizations with active transformation, you will experience a deeper level of fulfillment. The ethical aspirations that inform veganism—such as compassion, justice, freedom, nonviolence, and self-determination—are the very same values that inspire us to help humans. You will see this more and more, and rejecting excuses will become easier. Wherever you are on your path, give yourself permission to be imperfect. When you fail, tell yourself you'll do better next time.

## The Way Forward

I don't think many people would dispute the premise that the world is in a sorry state. It seems there's never been a time when we haven't had war or extreme poverty or mass injustice, and we could reasonably argue these blights are worse now than ever before. The number of animals we kill for food, for instance, is astronomical, and there are more humans enslaved today than at any time in our history. Violence has become normalized.

But we're beginning to see connections in how our treatment of others impacts us all—how those who abuse animals also hurt humans, how sexist people also have racist tendencies, how the slaughter of African elephants for ivory funds terrorism, how even a lack of compassion can adversely affect one's health. An injustice that doesn't hurt you likely helps you, and it's not always as apparent as a White person getting preferential treatment over a person of color. (I am reminded of a video demonstrating how one teacher explained privilege to his students by having them try to throw wadded-up paper into a recycle bin at the front of the class while they remained at their desks. Most of those seated in the first row easily sank the paper into the bin, while students toward the back rarely hit the target and complained about the game being unfair. "The closer you were to the recycling bin, the better your odds," the teacher said. "This is what privilege looks like," because the people seated in the front didn't consider how difficult it would be for the people in the back—or didn't care.) When those with privilege remain silent about those without, we become complicit in their oppression, just as a meat-eater is complicit in the death of the animal he or she is consuming.

If you aspire to live in a world without suffering, discrimination, or oppression, why not begin the cultural shift right now? Can you agree that "cruelty free" means more than just avoiding products with animal ingredients? Can you make a personal commitment to be more mindful of your consumer choices, taking into consideration the lives of workers who sow, tend, and harvest our fruits, vegetables, legumes, and grains; the Indigenous peoples on whose land palm oil is produced; and the children forced to toil in cocoa plantations?

Going vegan is a great first step, but it's only the beginning. Homophobia, racism, sexism, transphobia, and ableism—like speciesism—are learned beliefs we acquire through social programming, and that means society can unlearn these negative thought patterns. The first challenge is acknowledging they exist in the first place. Sadly, many people believe that racism is something that disappeared with silent movies. It is critical that we own up to the behaviors we use to marginalize others. Acknowledgement can aid healing and helps us become agents of change.

Children play a critical role in this change as they become the next generation of community leaders and society influencers. So let's discuss social injustices with kids. Just as we'd tell them where a "chicken nugget" comes from, let's not be afraid to talk to them about race, to teach them how to recognize sexism, and to openly discuss White privilege. Teaching them tolerance and equality at home and in schools is probably the most important thing we can do to ensure a genuine, lasting transformation. And let's end the destructive, culturally imposed stereotypes that boys must never show emotion; that aggression is a sign of strength; and that "real men" eat meat, are only attracted to women, and must be competitive.

Don't think of what I am suggesting as revolutionary (I'm hardly the first person to encourage a more holistic view of compassion); think of this as *evolutionary*. If humanity hopes to flourish, if we'd like the legacy we leave to future generations to be justice and peace, then the task before us is to evolve into a more conscious species, fully awake to the consequences our fears and habits have on humans, other animals, and the environment.

Look at it this way: The unsustainable, unhealthy way most humans live now is only making us sick and miserable. Isn't it about time we try a different approach? I'm asking us to create a vegan ecosystem in which we can grow a thriving new world. I'm not naive; I understand that what I'm seeking seems unattainable, and it's not a goal we will see realized anytime soon. But can we at least begin to take into account the lives of everyone, regardless of their species, race, color, gender, sexual identity, or other social construct? Knowing what we know now, we can make choices that benefit not only ourselves, but those with whom we share this planet.

That is, after all, what it means to live a vegan ethic.

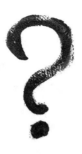

## Chapter 6

# Q & A

Every vegan gets questions about their veganism and their views about animal rights. Sometimes these questions are prompted by genuine curiosity; other times, they come from antagonists who are trying to prove the other person is wrong or from conflicted people hoping to resolve the moral dilemma of eating and using animals. Here are a dozen of the most common questions not addressed elsewhere in this book and information to help you answer them.

### 1. Could a vegan diet solve world hunger?

A frequent argument in favor of veganism is that because much of the world's water, grain, and arable land are used to raise and kill animals for food, no one on Earth would go hungry if those resources were instead used to feed humans a strictly plant-based diet. While as an ethical vegan I would love to endorse this reasoning, most food justice advocates would probably tell you that the reality is far more complex. They would point out, for example, that there is currently enough food produced to feed some 12 billion people, yet more than 900 million people are unable to meet their daily nutritional needs.

Part of the problem lies in global economics: those who are poor today and cannot afford to buy food would still be without the ability to pay for food in our vegan utopia. Another problem is how food is distributed, with many people simply not having access to what they require. Governments factor in here, too, as greed and corruption impact who gets what. Moreover, the food system is structured to maximize profit, with just a handful of companies controlling the majority of the food supply.

That said, I believe veganism is the best choice for the planet. Though a vegan world would still be faced with food inequities, diets based on plants rather than animals is a much more efficient, not to mention compassionate, system.

## 2. What would happen to all the farmed animals if everyone went vegan?

This is another one of those questions omnivores pose to try to make vegans feel guilty and to justify their own meat-eating. Keep in mind that the overwhelming majority of animals killed for food are essentially human creations living in factory farms and in only a few ways physically resemble their non-domesticated counterparts. In nature, for example, turkeys can fly and mate on their own, unlike turkeys in animal agriculture, where they have been bred to grow so heavy so quickly that they can barely stand after a few months.

If demand for meat, eggs, and dairy products ceased, the population of cows, chickens, pigs, and other animals bred and raised for food would certainly dwindle. But such a change would happen gradually: as more and more people adopt veganism, animal agriculture would have no choice but to artificially inseminate fewer and fewer animals. The land previously used for factory farms and feed crops would revert to nature, where wildlife would once again flourish.

Most of the animal species we've bred for food would probably thrive, though in much lower numbers. Chickens, pigs, turkeys, sheep, and fishes would find a natural balance in a world without animal slaughter. Cows are another matter. They were domesticated from a species of wild ox known as the auroch that roamed parts of Africa, Asia, and Europe before humans finally hunted them to extinction in the seventeenth century. While it is possible modern-day cows could survive in the wild, it's also possible they could die off. Currently, they just live to be killed.

However nature sorts things out, it will be a healthier and more peaceful planet for everyone.

### 3. Isn't "humane meat" a good option?

No one wants to feel like they are contributing to someone's misery, so it's only natural that a meat-eater would want to find the "kindest" way possible to continue their habit of consuming animals. Animal agribusiness capitalizes on this with a variety of "humane" alternatives to factory-farmed meat, and you see the results in grocery stores and restaurants: labels such as "free range," "organic," "cage free," and "certified humane" give consumers the impression that the animals lived a happy life with access to the outdoors and had "only one bad day."

Much of the cruelty of meat, eggs, and dairy, however, has been built right into the animal. Even chickens raised on pastures have been bred to grow at an abnormally fast rate, leading to crippling leg injuries and heart failure, and cows used in the organic dairy industry—just like those in large-scale farms—have been so relentlessly manipulated for maximum milk production that their udders become infected, yet cows on organic dairies may not receive antibiotics to ease their suffering. Moreover, these cows are still impregnated and their babies are taken away at birth.

Chickens in the egg industry, meanwhile, don't fare any better. "Cage free" eggs, for example, usually come from thousands of hens who are crowded into large, filthy sheds with no access to sunshine or fresh air. And whatever the label, male chicks are deemed useless, so millions of them are ground up or otherwise disposed of like garbage every year.

No matter how they are raised, nearly all animals used for food end up transported in cramped trucks to exactly the same slaughterhouses used by factory farms, where they are hung upside down and their throats are cut, often while they are fully conscious and fighting to escape. All these animals want to live, and there is nothing humane about their deaths.

### 4. Many Indigenous peoples, such as the Inuit and Tibetans, rely on animals for protein. Would an ethical vegan have a problem with this?

Few ethical vegans take issue with circumstances where people eat animals because their survival depends on it. The Inuit inhabit a remote corner of the globe, and the subsistence hunting and fishing they practice is clearly not for recreation. The same goes for Tibetans, who live on a high, cold plateau on which almost nothing edible grows—save for some grass and shrubs that yaks seem to enjoy. Tibetans in turn eat yaks.

While it would be ideal if all cultures could be vegan, I think our time is better spent trying to educate the 99.9 percent of the population who have no excuses at all for eating animals than to criticize a small community of people trying to survive amid harsh conditions.

### 5. Isn't veganism more expensive than eating animals?

This is one of those questions that even vegans argue about. While a diet of grains, beans, vegetables, fruits, and nuts would in theory be cheaper than eating meat, eggs, and dairy products, in practice, few vegans eat only whole foods. Because our taste buds have been accustomed to eating animals, vegans often enjoy so-called "mock meats"—such as burgers, "chicken" strips, bacon, and ribs made from plant-based ingredients—that approximate the texture and flavor of cooked meat. These can be a lot more expensive than their animal-based counterparts (which are priced lower in part due to government subsidies).

Produce is expensive, but omnivores eat fruits and veggies, too, so that shouldn't be a factor when comparing the cost of vegan versus omni diets.

A major factor that is often overlooked, however, is the lack of access to vegan foods in some neighborhoods. In a typical low-income community, you will find a variety of fast-food restaurants and markets that sell cheap animal-based products, but there's often a dearth of fruit and vegetable options. Residents of these communities may be single parents, for example, and/or work multiple jobs to keep food on the table. Moreover, they may be forced to rely on public transportation. So, for a consumer in this community to eat a vegan diet, she or he may have to take several buses to and from another city to buy fresh produce and other plant-based foods. All this adds significant cost to a grocery budget. Some bus lines also limit the number of bags a rider can bring onto the bus, creating another burden. (Please keep all these in mind when you hear someone say it's easy for anyone to be vegan.)

The bottom line is that buying only unprocessed foods in bulk may be cheaper than buying meat, eggs, and dairy foods, but few vegans actually shop that way—assuming they even have access to it. At the same time, we should not overlook how a vegan diet benefits our healthcare bills!

## 6. Don't plants feel pain?

Here's a you're-no-better-than-I-am argument popular among omnivores. It's an idea that's been around since at least 1973, when the bestselling, New Age-y book *The Secret Life of Plants* claimed that fruits, vegetables, flowers, and trees were sentient beings.

From an evolutionary perspective, the evidence against plants feeling pain is strong, since plants have no ability to move out of harm's way. Recent research has indicated that plants respond to the sound of insects munching on their leaves, but that's a long way from saying they actually experience pain. For that, most biologists agree, plants would need to possess sensory organs and a nervous system.

None of this is to imply that plants are not extraordinary organisms. They have a remarkable ability to adapt to their environment and find nourishment from a fixed position. There's just nothing to suggest they feel pain. Animals, on the other hand, absolutely do.

To the person who tries to justify their meat-eating by claiming plants feel pain, remind them that 70 percent of crops go to feed farmed animals, so if they truly care about plants, not eating animals is the best way to ensure their safety.

## 7. Don't animals raised for meat benefit by being protected from predators and receiving medical care?

First of all, farmed animals are not protected; indeed, they are preyed upon by one of the world's deadliest predators—humans. Even cows and hens exploited for their milk and eggs are eventually killed once their bodies are "spent" from exploitation. As for the "medical care" they receive, agribusiness views animals as commodities. Any medical treatment administered is meant to keep an animal healthy long enough to kill him or her. Farmers also give animals liberal amounts of antibiotics to promote growth and compensate for the unsanitary conditions commonly found in confinement. It's all in the name of profit, not compassion.

## 8. Why do some people reject cruelty to animals while others don't?

As we consider the many ways humans exploit nonhuman animals, we are apt to question what's going on here. Why is society so entrenched in using animals? Advocates of animal liberation ask that, and they decide to reject such abuse. But they represent only a very small percentage of the public. What about the rest of us?

One theory I am especially drawn to has been proposed by Dr. Lori Marino and Michael Mountain. Lori is a biopsychologist and science director at the Nonhuman Rights Project, and Michael is an activist and one of the founders of Best Friends Animal Society. Their hypothesis is actually pretty simple: Humans are afraid of death. We react to that fear by thinking of ourselves as being qualitatively different from other animals, and we express that difference by treating animals as resources— lesser beings separate from ourselves.

Their idea is based on the work of researchers and authors, notably social anthropologist Ernest Becker, who popularized Terror Management Theory (TMT), which asserts that much of human behavior is motivated by our anxiety about personal mortality. According to TMT, humans respond by creating religions and looking to culture to find meaning in life.

But we also transfer our existential terror onto animals, say Lori and Michael. While it's true that other animals experience terror when confronted by death, they say, for us humans it's a lifelong obsession. We think far into the future about our impending demise, and that curses us with a chronic level of anxiety. We see animals die, and we are so terrified by the thought of death that we convince ourselves we are not animals. We tell ourselves that humans are superior to (other) animals and that they exist for our benefit—a notion that dates back at least to ancient Greece. We convince ourselves we have a soul, and they don't, and this kind of thinking leads to devastating consequences for animals, as we justify using them as food sources, test subjects, and objects for entertainment. It's our attempt to exert control over the natural world and our animal nature. We treat some animals better because we've come to look upon them as part of the human "in-group" and consider them family members.

## 9. Doesn't eating plants mean vegans are exploiting honeybees?

Insects, birds, and mammals pollinate most of our food crops, and honey producers want consumers to believe that honey is simply a byproduct of the pollination provided by honeybees. But honeybees are not as good at pollinating as many truly wild bees, such as bumblebees and carpenter and digger bees. These bees do not produce large amounts of honey, however, making it not worth the time to steal their honey. As a result, farmers continue to rely on factory-farmed honeybees for pollination, thus supporting a multimillion-dollar honey industry, which most vegans do not support. In the end, it's another no-win situations for vegans: there is almost no way to eliminate all animal exploitation from our lives.

## 10. What is the vegan position on pests? Even organic farms use methods like importing ladybugs to kill insects that eat crops. And termites, cockroaches, and rats can bring disease or make a home uninhabitable. Isn't any argument that differentiates animals into two categories (OK to kill/not OK to kill) undermining a vegan ethic?

A vegan ethic dictates that we should do our best not to harm anyone, and that includes "pests." I don't have a problem with ladybugs eating other insects, since that's how they survive and it's much better than using pesticides on plants. But there are some cases in which insects pose a real threat to our welfare or safety or that of companion animals, and under such circumstances we may have to kill fleas, termites, and other tiny creatures. It's one of those compromises vegans regrettably have to make sometimes.

But before things reach that point, we should take measures to prevent an invading horde by keeping kitchens spotlessly clean and using elements such as peppermint oil on windowsills to deter ants. Cockroaches, meanwhile, can't stand the smell of bay leaves (dry or fresh). Patch holes in walls and screens to keep rodents outside. Build a fake wasp nest (look it up online) in areas frequented by wasps; these insects are territorial and won't build a nest if they believe other wasps have already established themselves in the area. Make sure companion animals get regular flea and tick treatments. For those animals and insects who do get inside, there are non-lethal traps that allow you to take a mouse or rat to a field or carry an insect outdoors. You'll find plenty of advice about this topic on the Internet.

### 11. Isn't eating animals a personal choice?

The often-used rationale that eating animals is a personal choice assumes there is no victim. But a "personal choice" would affect only the person making the decision, and a choice to eat animals has consequences that reach far beyond the decision-maker. It affects animals who have no say in the matter, and it contributes to environmental destruction on a massive scale.

Implied in this excuse is an entreaty for vegans to leave meat-eaters alone; indeed, meat-eaters will sometimes add "I respect your food choices, so please respect mine." We have no obligation to respect a choice that hurts others.

Although most people consider what they eat to be a private matter, when they are eating someone else, it clearly crosses the line into non-personal territory. Picking out a book to read is a personal choice. Deciding to consume animals and support animal agriculture impacts everyone. A person's "right" to eat whatever they want ends where another's life begins.

### 12. Aren't more animals killed while harvesting crops than in slaughterhouses?

Here is yet another argument that meat-eaters offer to both assuage their guilt and try to make vegans regret their plant-based diets. Regrettably, some animals are indeed killed during industrialized crop harvesting. How many are killed, however, remains a mystery. In 2003, Steven Davis, an animal science professor at Oregon State University, looked at previous studies of mouse populations in fields and found that they dropped from 25 mice per hectare before harvesting to 5 per hectare after harvesting. Extrapolating from this data, Davis deduced that 10 animals per hectare are killed from crop farming each year. The problem with this conclusion is that no one can say if the animals were actually killed by harvesting machines or simply left the now-denuded field for better cover, such as a nearby forest.

With some 70 billion land animals butchered for human consumption worldwide every year, slaughterhouses remain the number-one place for killing animals—unless you consider the commercial fishing industry, which kills as many as 3 trillion fishes a year (as discussed in Chapter 1). Like the argument that plants feel pain, remember that most of the crops in the world are grown to feed farmed animals, not humans, so if someone is genuinely concerned about the deaths of field animals, they should go vegan.

# Appendix A: Ten Ways You Can Help Animals

1.  Go vegan. (See Appendix B.)
2.  Adopt companion animals from shelters—never buy from pet stores.
3.  Make sure the cosmetics and household products you use are not tested on animals.
4.  Write a letter to the editor of your local paper about an animal issue currently in the news.
5.  Include a signature line in your email that links to one of your favorite vegan recipes or animal rights videos. You can also add an inspiring quotation.
6.  Ask your school cafeteria or favorite non-vegan restaurant to offer (more) plant-based dishes.
7.  Contact a local animal shelter or sanctuary and ask about volunteering.
8.  Change the message people hear when they leave a message on your phone to one that advocates for animals.
9.  Redirect gifts. Instead of receiving birthday presents, ask friends and family to donate to your local animal shelter or other nonprofit organizations that work on behalf of animals.
10. Share this book with someone.

# Appendix B: Ten Ways to Make Veganism Easier

1. Take it one step at a time. If going vegan overnight seems daunting, make small changes and gradually adopt a vegan ethic by replacing animal-based foods in your meals with plant-based foods over time. For example, use almond milk instead of cow's milk the first week. The next week, replace the meat on your plate with a meat alternative such as a veggie burger, or simply add more vegetables and fruit to your meal. Soon you will have crowded animals right out of your diet—then you can start replacing leather and wool items from the closet. And so on.

2. Make progress—not perfection—your goal.

3. Eat more fruits and veggies at each meal. These are not only healthy, but they'll make you feel fuller.

4. Pick up a comprehensive vegan cookbook and learn to make at least three or four dishes you really enjoy, including comfort foods.

5. Give yourself extra time in the kitchen when you begin cooking vegan—preparing meals may take a little longer at first.

6. Discover the wonder of shopping at Asian markets, which are filled with vegan foods and ingredients.

7. When going to a non-vegan gathering, such as holiday dinners, bring a vegan dish. Not only will you be guaranteed to have at least one meal you can eat, but you can share it with others and impress them with how delicious veganism can be.

8. Get involved with a local vegan group, where you can meet like-minded people, share recipes, and feel supported.

9. Find one or two restaurants in your area that serve vegan-friendly dishes, so you have a place to dine on days you

don't feel like cooking. If you're not sure what vegan entrées your favorite restaurant offers, ask them. You'll be surprised how many non-vegan meals can be made vegan!

10. Keep your pantry and fridge stocked with essential ingredients, such as beans (dry or canned), grains (rice, flour, and quinoa), pasta, tofu, nuts, fresh produce, nutritional yeast, cooking oil, vegetable stock, soy or nut milk, agave, egg replacer, and seasonings. With these staples on hand, you'll be prepared to make a wide assortment of meals.

# Appendix C: Ten Ways You Can Encourage Someone Else to Go Vegan

1. Take them to visit a sanctuary for farmed animals.

2. Invite them to a vegan potluck or other vegan-related event.

3. Watch a video such as *Blackfish, Cowspiracy, Earthlings, The Ghosts in Our Machine, Food Inc., Live and Let Live,* or *Vegucated* together—and then discuss it.

4. Give them a copy of your favorite vegan cookbook and encourage them to try a recipe.

5. Bring them a delicious, home-cooked vegan meal.

6. Resist the urge to preach—no one likes a pushy vegan; instead, lead by example. Emphasize the benefits of being vegan rather than whatever challenges you may face.

7. Donate copies of your favorite vegan cookbooks and animal rights books to your local library.

8. Ask family and friends to be vegan on your birthday or for a day in lieu of holiday gifts.

9. Treat them to lunch or dinner at your favorite vegan restaurant.

10. Go grocery shopping with them, encouraging them to try new fruits and veggies and showing them how many plant-based foods and household products not tested on animals are available.

For more advice on vegan advocacy, read *Striking at the Roots: A Practical Guide to Animal Activism.*

# Appendix D: Ten Ways You Can Help Humanity

1. Never tolerate sexism, racism, homophobia, bullying, or any other forms of discrimination. If you're in the company of someone who uses a homophobic slur or tells a racist joke, for example, speak up and let them know how you feel.

2. Write to a prisoner of conscience, such as someone incarcerated for social justice or animal activism. Visit www.freedom-now.org/a-guide-to-writing-prisoners-of-conscience or www.directaction.info/prisoners.htm for more information. Of course, *any* prisoner, regardless of his or her crime, appreciates getting mail.

3. Do not buy chocolate sourced from the worst forms of child labor, including slavery. (See www.foodispower.org/chocolate-list)

4. Buy organic when you can, which helps farm workers a bit, as organic produce is not doused with chemicals.

5. Pass onto children respect for other cultures, respect for women, respect for other races, respect for anyone who is considered "different," and respect for themselves.

6. Get over any belief you may have that we live in a post-racial society. As much as we may not want to admit it, racism is everywhere, and Whites will never be part of restorative justice by thinking race has nothing to do with White police officers killing Black men, women, and children or by calling yourself "colorblind" (an ableist term when not referring to vision impairment).

7. Consider adopting a child.

8. Arrange to donate your body to science. This not only benefits humans, but it helps offset the use of animals for medical research.

9. Redirect gifts. Instead of receiving birthday presents, ask friends and family to donate money to nonprofit organizations that work on behalf of humans.

10. Donate vegan food to a local food bank. (See www.foodispower.org/donating-food-takes-thought)

# Appendix E: Twelve Famous (and Not-So-Famous) Quotations

The vegan and animal liberation movements are filled with inspiring quotations from notable writers, activists, and other public figures. Some utterances can indeed be linked to the person quoted, while others cannot. (Case in point: A famous remark attributed to Abraham Lincoln—"I am in favor of animal rights as well as human rights. That is the way of a whole human being"—has been roundly debunked as apocryphal.) Following are a dozen quotations, where each came from, and a bit about the person associated with it. I present these quotations not because they are well-known—indeed, many are not—but because they resonate with the themes in this book.

> *At last poor Wat was found, as he there lay,*
> *By Huntsmen, which came with their Dogs that way*
> *Whom seeing, he got up, and fast did run,*
> *Hoping some ways the Cruel Dogs to shun;*
> *But they by Nature had so quick a Sent,*
> *That by their Nose they Trac'd what way he went*
> —Margaret Cavendish (1623–73)

A member of England's nobility who spoke out against the popular aristocratic pastime of hunting, Margaret Cavendish, the Duchess of Newcastle-upon-Tyne, was a poet, a playwright, a scientist, a philosopher, and—with her views concerning humanity's exploitation of nature—a proto-ecofeminist. The above verse, extracted from her 1653 poem "The Hunting of the Hare," reflects Cavendish's distaste for blood sports. It concerns a hare named Wat, who is being tracked by dogs and is eventually killed. Animal welfare was considered a trivial issue during Cavendish's lifetime, yet she continued to denounce the accepted belief that animals existed merely as things to be exploited. Indeed, she directly challenged the French scientist René Descartes and his notion that animals were machines that felt nothing. As an early proponent of animal rights, Margaret Cavendish was a true pioneer.

*My food is not that of man; I do not destroy the lamb and the kid to glut my appetite; acorns and berries afford me sufficient nourishment.*
—Mary Wollstonecraft Shelley (1797–1851)

Although there's no evidence to suggest that English author, essayist, editor, and short-story and travel writer Mary Shelley ate a plant-based diet, she nevertheless created one of history's most memorable and enduring literary vegetarians: the humanoid Creature of her 1818 Gothic novel *Frankenstein*, who utters the words above. In the novel, Dr. Victor Frankenstein makes the Creature out of body parts gathered from graveyards, dissection labs, and slaughterhouses, thus creating a species that is both human and nonhuman. While Dr. Frankenstein is portrayed as a villain who eats meat and tortures live animals in the name of science, the Creature is at first a benevolent character, which extends to his vision for a peaceful vegetarian paradise, as he reveals when he proposes to Dr. Frankenstein that he create a partner for him. (For more insights on this, see *The Sexual Politics of Meat* by Carol J. Adams.)

*Vegetable diet and sweet repose. Animal food and nightmare. Pluck your body from the orchard; do not snatch it from the shambles. Without flesh diet there could be no blood-shedding war.*
—Louisa May Alcott (1832–88)

The acclaimed author of the autobiographical novel *Little Women* and many other works spent much of her childhood in Concord,

Massachusetts, where she came into contact with such freethinkers as Henry David Thoreau, Ralph Waldo Emerson, and Margaret Fuller. Although not a strict vegetarian like her father, Amos Bronson Alcott, Louisa used vegetarian images in her writing to advance the cause of women's rights and promote nonviolence. In addition to being an author, she was an abolitionist (her family's home was a stop on the Underground Railroad), a champion of social reform, and a nurse in the US Civil War. The quotation here comes from *Louisa May Alcott, Little Women: Letters from the House of Alcott,* published in 1914. ("Shambles" is an archaic term for slaughterhouse or meat market.)

*Now nearly all agree that the lower animals have certain rights, as inalienable as those of man to life, liberty and the pursuit of happiness.*
—Caroline Earle White (1833–1916)

Born into a distinguished Philadelphia family of abolitionists and suffragists, Caroline Earle White was the founder of three of Pennsylvania's most noteworthy animal organizations and a founding member of the American Humane Society. In 1866, she created a Philadelphia chapter of the American Society for the Prevention of Cruelty to Animals, but gender politics of the day excluded her from an official position, so three years later she founded the Women's Pennsylvania Society for the Prevention of Cruelty to Animals (WPSPCA), which opened the nation's first animal shelter (prior to this, homeless animals were simply killed) and operates today as the Women's Humane Society. White founded the American Anti-Vivisection Society (AAVS) in 1883, and in an early example of leafleting for animals, AAVS passed out millions of pamphlets at the 1893 Chicago World's Fair exposing the issue of pets stolen for research. Although White's quotation, which comes from her 1893 report to the

Board of WPSPCA, uses the term "lower animals," we must remember that her words are the product of an earlier era and that she was demonstrating compassion for beings regardless of their abilities.

*I was a cannibal for twenty-five years. For the rest I have been a vegetarian.*
—George Bernard Shaw (1856–1950)

Irish playwright, essayist, and journalist George Bernard Shaw may be best remembered for his writing (he was awarded the Nobel Prize for Literature in 1925), but he spoke out against many forms of animal cruelty, including blood sports and vivisection. He was also a vegetarian at a time when the prevailing view was that one simply *had* to eat meat to survive; indeed, some of Shaw's contemporaries suggested it was only a secret consumption of liver that kept him alive. After doctors advised him against his vegetarian diet, Shaw wrote to *The London Daily Chronicle*: "My will contains directions for my funeral, which will be followed not by mourning coaches, but by herds of oxen, sheep, swine, flocks of poultry, and a small travelling aquarium of live fish, all wearing white scarves in honour of the man who perished rather than eat his fellow-creatures." His quotation first appeared in *The Candid Friend* (May 1901).

*The butcher with his bloody apron incites bloodshed, murder. Why not? From cutting the throat of a young calf to cutting the throat of our brothers and sisters is but a step. While we are ourselves the living graves of murdered animals, how can we expect any ideal conditions on the earth?*
—Isadora Duncan (1877–1927)

Celebrated today as the creator of modern dance, Isadora Duncan was born in San Francisco and lived in Europe, where she developed a dancing style that focused on freedom and natural movement rather than the rigid technique common in ballet. She was renowned both for her performances and her nonconformist lifestyle—she was openly bisexual and had two children out of wedlock—and established several dancing schools. Though not strict about her vegetarianism (her diet may have been due to economic circumstances rather than ethics), Duncan boasted that "the children of my schools were all vegetarians, and grew strong and beautiful on a vegetable and fruit diet." She wrote about her vegetarianism in her 1927 autobiography *My Life*, from which this quotation is extracted.

*I have no objection to vivisection, provided the vivisectors experiment on themselves.*
—Lizzy Lind-af-Hageby (1878–1963)

Swedish-born Emilie Augusta Louise "Lizzy" Lind-af-Hageby was a prominent feminist, peace activist, and animal rights advocate who became one of England's most vocal critics of vivisection. In 1902, she and another activist from Sweden, Leisa Katherine Schartau, enrolled at the London School of Medicine for Women to augment their anti-vivisectionist education. The following year they published *The Shambles of Science: Extracts from the Diary of Two Students of Physiology*, which documented the cruelty to animals they had witnessed, including the inhumane treatment of a little terrier by several researchers at University College London, who experimented on the dog multiple times without anesthesia, in violation of the 1876 Cruelty to Animals Act. The outrage that followed led to a political controversy known as the Brown Dog Affair. Her little-known quotation comes from a letter to the editor in the February 3, 1909, edition of *The New York Times*.

*Now at last I can look at you in peace; I don't eat you anymore.*
—Franz Kafka (1883–1924)

Born in Prague, capital of what is now the Czech Republic, German-language novelist and short-story writer Franz Kafka was fond of spinning tales from an animal's point of view. His best-known work, the 1912 novella *The Metamorphosis*, features a protagonist who wakes up to find he's been turned into an enormous insect. In other stories, such as "The New Advocate," "The Animal in the Synagogue," and "Investigations of a Dog," animals figure prominently or even serve as narrators. According to his friend Max Brod, Kafka, who had recently become a vegetarian, was visiting the aquarium in Berlin when he gazed at the fishes in a tank and addressed them directly with the above quotation. In 1937, Brod published *Franz Kafka, A Biography*, which includes this passage.

*May we keep our compassion alive by eating in such a way that reduces the suffering of living beings, stops contributing to climate change, and heals and preserves our precious planet.*
—Thich Nhat Hanh (1926–)

Zen Buddhist monk and devout vegan Thich Nhat Hanh has eloquently written and spoken so often about the link between diet and compassion that it's difficult to choose just one quotation from him. But I think this sentence, presented as a contemplation in his 2014 book *How to Eat*, beautifully represents the essence of what it means to live a vegan ethic. He left his native Vietnam in 1966 on a peace mission to meet with Martin Luther King, Jr, Pope Paul VI, and others, seeking an end to the war in his homeland. Because Nhat Hanh advocated peace and reconciliation rather than victory, the former government of South Vietnam barred his return, as did the Communists who assumed control after the war. He was forced to live in exile, mainly in

France, where he established a vegan monastic community called Plum Village. He is regarded as the founder of Engaged Buddhism, a movement through which practitioners use peaceful activism for the purpose of social reform. In 2005, Thich Nhat Hanh was allowed to return to Vietnam for a three-month teaching visit.

> *Kindness and compassion towards all living things is a mark of a civilized society. Conversely, cruelty, whether it is directed against human beings or against animals, is not the exclusive province of any one culture or community of people.*
>
> *Racism, economic deprival, dog fighting and cock fighting, bullfighting and rodeos are cut from the same fabric: violence.*
>
> *Only when we have become nonviolent towards all life will we have learned to live well ourselves.*

—Cesar Chavez (1927–93)

Born into a Mexican-American family in Arizona, Cesar Chavez was a farm worker, labor leader, and civil rights activist. Together with Dolores Huerta, in 1962 he co-founded the National Farm Workers Association, later becoming the United Farm Workers Union (UFW). His nonviolent campaigns agitating for workers' rights included a series of boycotts, marches, and hunger strikes that brought unprecedented protections for farm laborers. Chavez was also an ethical vegan who made the connection between speciesism and other forms of oppression. "Cesar took genuine pride in producing numerous converts to vegetarianism over the decades. You're looking at one of them," UFW president Arturo Rodriguez said in 1996. "He felt so strongly about it that sometimes I think he took as much personal satisfaction from converting people to vegetarianism as he did to trade unionism." His quotation is part of a letter he wrote to the organization Action for Animals on December 26, 1990.

*Whenever people say "We mustn't be sentimental" you can take it they are about to do something cruel. And if they add "We must be realistic" they mean they are going to make money out of it.*
—Brigid Brophy (1929–95)

Brigid Brophy was an English novelist, a social critic, and a crusader for many causes, including the rights of women and nonhuman animals. Her first novel, *Hackenfeller's Ape* (1953), concerns a scientist who risks his career to save an ape from being blasted on a one-way trip into outer space in the name of military advancement. In October 1965, *The Sunday Times* in London published her landmark essay "The Rights of Animals," which has led some scholars to pinpoint that year as the beginning of the modern animal rights movement. Brophy was also a vice president of the National Anti-Vivisection Society. Her quotation is from the 1985 anthology *Unlived Life: A Manifesto Against Factory Farming*, edited by Jon Wynne-Tyson.

*There can be no great triumph over racism without addressing capitalism, sexism, homophobia, transphobia, the environment that we live in, and the food that we consume. We have to recognize all of these connections.*
—Angela Davis (1944–)

Alabama native Angela Davis is a writer, educator, feminist, vegan, and civil rights activist and organizer who rose to prominence in the 1960s and 1970s as a member of the Student Nonviolent Coordinating Committee and the Black Panther Party. Organizing on behalf of three Black inmates on trial for murder, Davis ended up behind bars, charged with criminal conspiracy, kidnapping, and first-degree murder. A worldwide movement formed to free her from jail, and she was eventually cleared of all charges. Her concern for prisoners' rights led Davis to found Critical Resistance, a national organization dedicated to dismantling the prison industrial complex. Her comments above come from a speech she made during Angela Davis: A Lifetime of Revolution, an event honoring her at the University of Southern California on February 23, 2015.

# Appendix F: Resources

There are many resources available; this is just a very brief list.

## Animal Rights Groups

### *Australia*

Against Animal Cruelty Tasmania
www.aact.org.au

Animals Australia
www.animalsaustralia.org

Animal Liberation Victoria
www.alv.org.au

Edgar's Mission
http://edgarsmission.org.au

Humane Research Australia
www.humaneresearch.org.au

### *Canada*

Campaigns Against the Cruelty to Animals
www.catcahelpanimals.org

Canadian Animal Liberation Movement
www.calmaction.org

Canadian Voice for Animals
www.canadianvoiceforanimals.org

EarthSave Canada
www.earthsave.ca

Fur-Bearer Defenders
www.banlegholdtraps.com

Toronto Pig Save
www.torontopigsave.org

Toronto Vegetarian Association
www.veg.ca

Vancouver Humane Society
www.vancouverhumanesociety.bc.ca

ZooCheck
www.zoocheck.com

## *Europe*

Animal Aid
www.animalaid.org.uk

Animal Equality
www.animalequality.net

Animal Rights Action Network
www.aran.ie

Coalition to Abolish Animal Testing
www.ohsukillsprimates.com

Coalition to Abolish the Fur Trade
www.caft.org.uk

Cruelty Free International
www.crueltyfreeinternational.org

European Coalition to End Animal Experiments
www.eceae.org

League Against Cruel Sports
www.league.org.uk

Viva!
www.viva.org.uk

## New Zealand

Direct Animal Action
www.directanimalaction.org.nz

Farmwatch
www.farmwatch.org.nz

Greyhound Protection League of New Zealand
http://gplnz.org

New Zealand Anti-Vivisection Society
www.nzavs.org.nz

Save Animals From Exploitation
www.safe.org.nz

## South Africa

Beauty Without Cruelty South Africa
www.bwcsa.co.za

Seal Alert
https://sealalertsa.wordpress.com

## *United States*

Animal Legal Defense Fund
www.aldf.org

Animals & Society Institute
www.animalsandsociety.org

Beagle Freedom Project
www.beaglefreedomproject.org

Born Free USA
www.bornfreeusa.org

Compassionate Action for Animals
www.exploreveg.org

CompassionWorks International
www.cwint.org

Farm Animal Rights Movement
www.farmusa.org

Farm Sanctuary
www.farmsanctuary.org

Fish Feel
www.fishfeel.org

Food Empowerment Project
www.foodispower.org

Free from Harm
http://freefromharm.org

Mercy For Animals
www.mercyforanimals.org

Nonhuman Rights Project
www.nonhumanrightsproject.org

Sea Shepherd Conservation Society
www.seashepherd.org

SHARK
www.sharkonline.org

United Poultry Concerns
www.upc-online.org

Vegan Outreach
www.veganoutreach.org

VINE Sanctuary
www.bravebirds.org

A Well-Fed World
http://awfw.org

Woodstock Farm Sanctuary
http://woodstocksanctuary.org

## Books

### *For Activism*

*The Animal Activist's Handbook: Maximizing Our Positive Impact in Today's World*
Matt Ball and Bruce Friedrich

*Bleating Hearts: The Hidden World of Animal Suffering*
Mark Hawthorne

*Defiant Daughters: 21 Women on Art, Activism, Animals, and the Sexual Politics of Meat*
Edited by Kara Davis and Wendy Lee

*Entangled Empathy: An Alternative Ethic for Our Relationships with Animals*
Lori Gruen

*Ethics Into Action: Henry Spira and the Animal Rights Movement*
Peter Singer

*Growl: Life Lessons, Hard Truths, and Bold Strategies from an Animal Advocate*
Kim Stallwood

*In Defense of Animals: The Second Wave*
Edited by Peter Singer

*The Lines We Draw*
Sangamithra Iyer

*The Master Communicator's Handbook*
Teresa Erickson and Tim Ward

*Meat Market: Animals, Ethics, and Money*
Erik Marcus

*Move the Message: Your Guide to Making a Difference and Changing the World*
Josephine Bellaccomo

*Nature Ethics: An Ecofeminist Perspective*
Marti Kheel

*The Oxen at the Intersection: A Collision*
pattrice jones

*Sister Species: Women, Animals, and Social Justice*
Lisa Kimmerer

*Striking at the Roots: A Practical Guide to Animal Activism*
Mark Hawthorne

*Uncaged: Top Activists Share Their Wisdom on Effective Farm Animal Advocacy*
Ben Davidow

*We Animals*
Jo-Anne McArthur

## *For Support*

*Aftershock: Confronting Trauma in a Violent World: A Guide for Activists and Their Allies*
pattrice jones

*Animal Grace: Entering a Spiritual Relationship with Our Fellow Creatures*
Mary Lou Randour

*Healing Through the Dark Emotions: The Wisdom of Grief, Fear, and Despair*
Miriam Greenspan

*The Inner Art of Vegetarianism: Spiritual Practices for Body and Soul*
Carol J. Adams

*Striking at the Roots: A Practical Guide to Animal Activism*
Mark Hawthorne

*Vegan Freak: Being Vegan in a Non-Vegan World*
Bob and Jenna Torres

*Vegan's Daily Companion: 365 Days of Inspiration for Cooking, Eating, and Living Compassionately*
Colleen Patrick-Goudreau

### Cookbooks
You will find hundreds of titles online; these are just a few suggestions.

*Afro-Vegan: Farm-Fresh African, Caribbean, and Southern Flavors Remixed*
Bryant Terry

*Eat Like You Give a Damn*
Michelle Schwegmann and Josh Hooten

*Eat Vegan on $4 a Day: A Game Plan for the Budget-Conscious Cook*
Ellen Jaffe Jones

*The Joy of Vegan Baking*
Colleen Patrick-Goudreau

*One-Dish Vegan: More than 150 Soul-Satisfying Recipes for Easy and Delicious One-Bowl and One-Plate Dinners*
Robin Robertson

*Vegan for Her: The Woman's Guide to Being Healthy and Fit on a Plant-Based Diet*
Virginia Messina

*Vegan Planet: 400 Irresistible Recipes with Fantastic Flavors from Home and Around the World*
Robin Robertson

*Vegan with a Vengeance*
Isa Chandra Moskowitz

## Related to Veganism

*The 30-Day Vegan Challenge (New Edition): The Ultimate Guide to Eating Healthfully and Living Compassionately*
Colleen Patrick-Goudreau

*Always Too Much and Never Enough: A Memoir*
Jasmin Singer

*The Face on Your Plate: The Truth about Food*
Jeffrey Moussaieff Masson

*Healthy at 100: The Scientifically Proven Secrets of the World's Healthiest and Longest-Lived Peoples*
John Robbins

*How to Be Vegan: Tips, Tricks, and Strategies for Cruelty-Free Eating, Living, Dating, Travel, Decorating, and More*
Elizabeth Castoria

*It's Easy to Start Eating Vegan: A Step-by-Step Guide with Recipes*
Rebecca Gilbert

*Main Street Vegan: Everything You Need to Know to Eat Healthfully and Live Compassionately in the Real World*
Victoria Moran and Adair Moran

*Never Too Late to Go Vegan: The Over-50 Guide to Adopting and Thriving on a Plant-Based Diet*
Carol J. Adams, Patti Breitman, and Virginia Messina

*The Polar Bear in the Zoo: A Speculation*
Martin Rowe

*Sistah Vegan: Black Female Vegans Speak on Food, Identity, Health, and Society*
Edited by A. Breeze Harper

*The Ultimate Betrayal: Is There Happy Meat?*
Hope Bohanec

*The Ultimate Vegan Guide: Compassionate Living without Sacrifice*
Erik Marcus

*Vegan for Life: Everything You Need to Know to Be Healthy and Fit on a Plant-Based Diet*
Jack Norris and Virginia Messina

*Vegetarian Paris: The Complete Insider's Guide to the Best Veggie Food in Paris*
Aurelia d'Andrea

*Will's Red Coat*
Tom Ryan

# Magazines

Barefoot Vegan
www.barefootvegan.com

Chickpea
http://chickpeamagazine.com

Laika
www.laikamagazine.com

Satya
http://satyamag.com

Swell! Magazine
www.swellmagazine.com

The Vegan
www.vegansociety.com/resources/publications-video/vegan-magazine

T.O.F.U. Magazine
www.ilovetofu.ca

Vegan Health and Fitness
www.veganhealthandfitnessmag.com

Vegan Lifestyle Magazine
www.veganlifestylemagazine.com

Vegan Magazine
www.vegan-magazine.com

VegNews
http://vegnews.com

## Additional Online Resources

American Vegan Society
www.americanvegan.org

Animal Rights Meetups
www.meetup.com/topics/animalrights

Animal Visuals
www.animalvisuals.org

Black Lives Matter
http://blacklivesmatter.com

Black Women For Wellness
www.bwwla.org

Black Vegans Rock
www.blackvegansrock.com

Center for Farmworker Families
www.farmworkerfamily.org

Critical Resistance (works to end the prison industrial complex)
http://criticalresistance.org

Faunalytics (free research tools for animal advocates)
https://faunalytics.org

Food Fight! Grocery
www.foodfightgrocery.com

Herbivore Clothing
www.herbivoreclothing.com

House Rabbit Society
www.rabbit.org

HumanTrafficking.org

Institute for Humane Education
http://humaneeducation.org

Joyful Vegan
www.joyfulvegan.com

Kim Stallwood (independent animal rights scholar)
www.kimstallwood.com

Kimmela Center for Animal Advocacy
www.kimmela.org

The Last 1000 (documenting the remaining chimpanzees in US
research labs)
http://last1000chimps.com

Love 146 (works to end child exploitation and trafficking)
https://love146.org

National Women's Coalition Against Violence & Exploitation
(US)
http://nwcave.org

#Not1More
www.notonemoredeportation.com

Our Hen House
www.ourhenhouse.org

Queer Vegan Food
http://queerveganfood.com

Rabbit Advocacy Network
www.rabbitadvocacynetwork.org

SaveABunny
www.SaveABunny.org

Sentience South Africa
www.sentience.co.za

Sistah Vegan Project
http://sistahvegan.com

Striking at the Roots (blog on animal activism)
https://strikingattheroots.wordpress.com

The Thinking Vegan
http://thethinkingvegan.com

The Vegan Society (UK)
www.vegansociety.com

Vegan.com

Vegan Feminist Network
http://veganfeministnetwork.com

Vegan Mexican Food
www.veganmexicanfood.com

Vegan Street
www.veganstreet.com

We Animals
www.weanimals.org

World of Vegan
www.worldofvegan.com

# Notes

## Introduction

**...the population of Tibetan exiles around the world today is estimated to number about 150,000...** Edward Wong, "Tibetans in exile debate independence," *The New York Times*, November 21, 2008.

## Chapter 1: On Animal Rights

**[Human is] a biological term.** I am indebted to biopsychologist and animal-personhood advocate Dr. Lori Marino for pointing out this important distinction.

**...in the United States, overall consumption of meat from cows, chickens, and fishes dropped 10 percent...** www.msnbc .com/msnbc/the-decline-red-meat-america

**...after being chained for months in a wooden crate so they can't use their muscles...** The American Veal Association has voted to phase out crates on all farms by 2017.

**Factory-farmed pigs have been so genetically altered...** Nathanael Johnson, "Swine of the Times: The making of the modern pig," *Harper's Magazine*, May 2006.

**Some former slaughterhouse workers...** Mark H. Bernstein, *Without a Tear: Our Tragic Relationship with Animals*, University of Illinois Press, 2004, page 97.

**Recent research has found that fishes...** Culum Brown, "Fish intelligence, sentience and ethics," *Animal Cognition*, January 2015, Volume 18, Issue 1.

**...with the commercial fishing industry catching as many as 3 trillion fishes a year.** http://fishcount.org.uk/

**...experiments show crustaceans...** http://blogs.nature.com/ news/2013/08/experiments-reveal-that-crabs-and-lobsters-feel-pain.html

**"The dolphin's life in a pool..."** William Johnson, *The Rose-*

*Tinted Menagerie*, Heretic Books, 1990, page 182.

**...it's important to note that zoos are traditionally tied to colonialism...** See *Reading Zoos: Representations of Animals in Captivity* by Randy Malamud, NYU Press, 1998.

**One study showed that children even demonstrated a "negative learning outcome"...** See www.captiveanimals.org/news/2014/09/zoos-neither-educate-empower-children-newly-published-research-suggests

## Chapter 2: On Veganism

**...but they are embracing a vegan ethic by boycotting marine parks...** See for example Laura McVicker, "SeaWorld attendance and revenue continues to decline," NBCSanDiego.com, February 26, 2015; Natalie DiBlasio, "Celebs join the fight against animal-tested cosmetics," USAToday.com, March 13, 2013; and Clint Jasper, "Lower production, changing fashions drive down sales of woollen clothing," abc.net.au, December 4, 2014.

**Donald Watson, one of the founders of The Vegan Society, put it this way...** https://www.vegansociety.com/sites/default/files/DW_Interview_2002_Unabridged_Transcript.pdf

**...but those who go vegan for the animals are less likely to abandon their diet...** Alexandra Sifferlin, "These Vegans Are More Likely to Stick With It," Time.com, April 6, 2015.

**The big one seems to be cheese.** This may be because cheese contains a protein called casein. When the human body digests casein, it produces casomorphins, which have an opiate-like effect on humans. Because cheese is denser than milk, the casein is more heavily concentrated, meaning that eating cheese produces a larger amount of casomorphins in the body compared to eating other dairy products.

**Vegan dietitians say a couple servings...** See http://jacknor-risrd.com/response-to-not-soy-fast/

## Chapter 3: On Human Rights

**According to some scholars...** See, for instance, *The Longest Struggle: Animal Advocacy from Pythagoras to PETA* by Norm Phelps (2007), and *A Companion to Gender History*, edited by Teresa A. Meade and Merry E. Wiesner-Hanks (2004)—just two examples.

**The theories of Friedrich Engels...** See *The Origin of the Family, Private Property and the State* by Friedrich Engels (1884). Not all of Engels' speculations have found favor with modern historians, but he was an outspoken proponent of gender equality.

**Joan Dunayer observes...** See Joan Dunayer, "Sexist Words, Speciesist Roots" in *Animals and Women: Feminist Theoretical Explorations*, edited by Carol J. Adams and Josephine Donovan, Duke University Press, 1995.

**Breaking away from this latter tradition is the ecofeminist movement...** See "Ecofeminism Revisited: Rejecting Essentialism and Re-Placing Species in a Material Feminist Environmentalism" by Greta Gaard, *Feminist Formations*, Volume 23, Number 2, Summer 2011, pages 26–53.

**As pattrice put it...** See https://www.youtube.com/watch?v=x0FjZQC8gcs

**...the average life expectancy of a farm worker in the US is only 49 years?** www.ufw.org/_page.php?menu=research&inc=history/12.html

**According to one of the rare studies...** http://cironline.org/reports/female-workers-face-rape-harassment-us-agriculture-industry-4798

**By one estimate, 80 percent of women and girls...** http://fusion.net/story/17321/is-rape-the-price-to-pay-for-migrant-women-chasing-the-american-dream/

**"When they resisted, they were killed."** http://agriworkers.org/system/files/so-2012june-therealtrespassers.pdf

**According to a BBC report...** Joao Fellet, "High murder rates blight Brazil's indigenous communities," BBC.com, February 28, 2014.

**Nearly 300 children are killed...** http://humantraffickingsearch.net/wp/child-forced-labor-part-ii-agriculture-in-the-americas/

**...where the sick are thrown overboard and the defiant are beheaded...** Ian Urbina, "'Sea Slaves': Forced Labor for Cheap Fish," *The New York Times*, July 27, 2015.

**Children growing up in homes with animal abuse and domestic violence...** As we consider the behavior we pass along to children as normal, let's not overlook the violent language many men use to describe their interactions with women: "hit on," "knock up," "hit that," etc.

**Author and activist Suzanne Pharr...** Suzanne Pharr, *Homophobia: A Weapon of Sexism*, Chardon Press, 1997, page 48.

**Kimberlé Crenshaw observes that shelters...** Kimberlé Williams Crenshaw, "Mapping the Margins: Intersectionality, Identity Politics, and Violence against Women of Color," *Stanford Law Review*, Volume 43, Number 6, July 1991.

**It wasn't until 2013, when I heard pattrice jones speak at an animal rights conference in Luxembourg...** You can watch pattrice's talk here: http://blog.bravebirds.org/archives/1553

**Indeed, there are now more Black men in prison, on probation, or on parole...** Max Ehrenfreund, "There's a disturbing truth to John Legend's Oscar statement about prisons and slavery," *Washington Post*, February 23, 2015.

**And with many more people of color than Whites being made felons...** See Michelle Alexander's 2010 book *The New Jim Crow: Mass Incarceration in the Age of Colorblindness*.

**Social activist Angela Davis observes...** Angela Davis, "Masked Racism: Reflections on the Prison Industrial Complex," *ColorLines*, Fall 1998.

**In Arlington, Virginia, for example, two 10-year-old boys...** Anjetta McQueen, "Youth violence down, suspensions on rise,"

Associated Press, April 12, 2000.

**According to the US Department of Education Office for Civil Rights...** http://ocrdata.ed.gov/Downloads/CRDC-School-Discipline-Snapshot.pdf

**Meanwhile, LGBTQ youth represent just 5 to 7 percent...** Jerome Hunt and Aisha C. Moodie-Mills, "The Unfair Criminalization of Gay and Transgender Youth: An Overview of the Experiences of LGBT Youth in the Juvenile Justice System," Center for American Progress, June 2012.

**These students may be three times more likely...** Andrew Cray, Katie Miller, and Laura E. Durso, "Seeking Shelter: The Experiences and Unmet Needs of LGBT Homeless Youth," Center for American Progress, September 2013.

**Once suspended from school, there is an increased likelihood...** www.aclu.org/fact-sheet/what-school-prison-pipe line#4

**In India, children as young as four years old...** www.bbc.com/news/world-asia-india-25556965

**According to the Urban Institute...** http://money.cnn. com/2014/10/21/pf/labor-trafficking/

**Those who resist or don't "follow the rules" might be severely beaten or killed.** Theresa Fisher, "Victim of Sex Trafficking in U.S. Tells Her Story," Juvenile Justice Information Exchange (jjie.org), January 23, 2014.

**Women are enticed with offers of legitimate work...** www.soroptimist.org/trafficking/faq.html

**...women and girls account for 98 percent of those trafficked...** Stephanie Hepburn and Rita J. Simon, *Human Trafficking Around the World: Hidden in Plain Sight*, Columbia University Press, 2013, page 2.

**But at least one study, released in 2008...** Richard Curtis, Meredith Dank, Kirk Dombrowski, Bilal Khan, Melissa Labriola, Amy Muslim, Michael Rempel, and Karen Terry, "The Commercial Sexual Exploitation of Children in New York City,"

Report to the National Institute of Justice, New York, NY, Center for Court Innovation and John Jay College of Criminal Justice, September 2008.

**[LGBTQ] represent about 40 percent of homeless youth...** Laura E. Durso and Gary J. Gates, "Serving Our Youth: Findings from a National Survey of Service Providers Working with Lesbian, Gay, Bisexual, and Transgender Youth Who Are Homeless or at Risk of Becoming Homeless," The Williams Institute with True Colors Fund and The Palette Fund, July 2012.

**...some 26 percent of homeless LGBTQ youth have been kicked out of their homes because...** http://www.sdgln.com/news/2010/02/09/sex-trafficking-hits-san-diegos-lgbt-youths#sthash.0Rd4NAUe.dpbs

**According to statistics gathered by Thorn...** www.wearethorn.org/online-exploitation-child-sex-trafficking-escort-websites/?utm_source=tw&utm_medium=tweet&utm_campaign=blog

**(Amnesty International estimates the nation puts thousands of people to death each year.)** www.amnesty.org.uk/sites/default/files/death_sentences_and_executions_2014_en.pdf

**...blistering pain for up to two hours...** www.latimes.com/nation/nationnow/la-na-nn-arizona-execution-20140723-story.html

**"I feel my whole body burning."** http://nation.time.com/2014/01/10/oklahoma-convict-who-felt-body-burning-executed-with-controversial-drug

**Of the 35 prisoners the US executed in 2014...** www.death-penaltyinfo.org/execution-list-2014

**...researchers from Ohio State University found...** www.deathpenaltyinfo.org/node/476

**Latinos, meanwhile, are 1.4 times more likely...** Jason T. Carmichael, David Jacobs, Stephanie L. Kent, and Zhenchao Qian, "Who Survives on Death Row? An Individual and Contextual Analysis," *American Sociological Review*, Volume 72,

August 2007.

**...researchers in Louisiana concluded...** Frank R. Baumgartner and Tim Lyman, "Race-of-Victim Discrepancies in Homicides and Executions, Louisiana 1976–2015," *Loyola University of New Orleans Journal of Public Interest Law,* Fall 2015.

**Among the first capital offenses codified in the eighteenth century...** Stuart Banner, *The Death Penalty: An American History,* Harvard University Press, 2002, page 8.

**"a truly unfortunate episode in our history."** www.cbsnews.com/news/south-carolina-boy-executed-for-1944-murder-is-exonerated

**By one estimate, between 1877 and 1950...** Equal Justice Initiative, "Lynching in America: Confronting the Legacy of Racial Terror," February 2015.

**...many studies show it does not have any impact on crime rates...** M. Radelet and T. Lacock, "Do Executions Lower Homicide Rates?: The Views of Leading Criminologists," *Journal of Criminal Law and Criminology,* Volume 99, Number 2, 2009.

**"One argument for the death penalty is that it is a strong deterrent to murder..."** Jimmy Carter, "Show Death Penalty the Door," *Atlanta Journal-Constitution,* April 25, 2012.

## Chapter 4: On the Environment

**The role of meat, egg, and dairy foods in climate change has been quantified by a team of British researchers...** John Upton, "Going vegetarian can cut your diet's carbon footprint in half," Grist.org, June 27, 2014.

**...a 2014 study examining 25 years of data...** Robert B. Wielgus and Kaylie A. Peebles, "Effects of Wolf Mortality on Livestock Depredations," *PLOS One,* December 3, 2014.

**According to the Center for Biological Diversity...** www.biologicaldiversity.org/programs/public_lands/grazing

**Scientists estimate that if meat production continues to grow...** Brian Machovina, Kenneth J. Feeley, William J. Ripple,

"Biodiversity conservation: The key is reducing meat consumption," *Science of the Total Environment*, Volume 536, December 1, 2015.

**Researchers from the University of Minnesota...** Lara P. Clark, Dylan B. Millet, and Julian D. Marshall, "National Patterns in Environmental Injustice and Inequality: Outdoor NO$_2$ Air Pollution in the United States," *PLOS One*, April 15, 2014.

**...Robert D. Bullard observes...** Robert D. Bullard, "Confronting Environmental Racism in the Twenty-First Century," *Global Dialogue*, Volume 4, Number 1, Winter 2002.

**...Hurricane Katrina killed 1836 people...**www.datacenterresearch.org/data-resources/katrina/facts-for-impact/

**Most of the areas that were completely washed out...** Reilly Morse, "Environmental Justice through the Eye of Hurricane Katrina," Joint Center for Political and Economic Studies, Inc., Washington, DC, 2008.

**"Hurricane Katrina and its aftermath..."** Van Jones, "The New Environmentalists," *ColorLines*, Issue 39, July/August 2007.

**"To put it bluntly"** Van Jones, "The New Environmentalists," *ColorLines*, Issue 39, July/August 2007.

**"This country can save the polar bears and poor kids too."** Van Jones, *The Green Collar Economy: How One Solution Can Fix Our Two Biggest Problems*, HarperCollins, 2008, page 22.

**...some ecofeminists also refer to as the "logic of domination"...** For more on the logic of domination, see *Ecofeminist Philosophy: A Western Perspective on What It Is and Why It Matters* by Karen J. Warren (2000), and *Feminism and the Mastery of Nature* by Val Plumwood (2002), as well as the work of Greta Gaard and Lori Gruen.

**A 571-page scientific report...** United States Department of Agriculture, "Scientific Report of the 2015 Dietary Guidelines Advisory Committee," February 2015.

**It takes 450 gallons of water to produce a hamburger...** http://water.usgs.gov/edu/activity-watercontent.html

One gallon of cow's milk requires 880 gallons of water. http://environment.nationalgeographic.com/environment/freshwater/embedded-water/

Farmed animals account for at least 32,000 million tons of carbon dioxide per year... www.worldwatch.org/node/6294

Farmed animals are responsible for 65 percent of all emissions of nitrous oxide... www.fao.org/docrep/010/a0701e/a0701e00.htm

Each lactating cow used in the dairy industry produces about 150 pounds of manure a day... James M. MacDonald, Marc O. Ribaudo, Michael J. Livingston, Jayson Beckman, and Wen Huang, "Manure Use for Fertilizer and for Energy—Report to Congress," USDA Economic Research Service, June 2009.

...a vegan diet reduces his or her carbon emissions by 1.5 metric tons a year. www.newscientist.com/article/dn25795-going-vegetarian-halves-co2-emissions-from-your-food

Every second, 1.5 acres of rainforest are cleared. www.savetherainforest.org/savetherainforest_007.htm

Farmed animals and crops grown to feed them are the leading causes of rainforest destruction. www.fao.org/ag/magazine/0612sp1.htm

## Chapter 5: On a More Compassionate World

...as the late activist and author Norm Phelps observed... http://everydayutilitarian.com/essays/one-struggle-one-fight

...Black communities, to whom even the word "animal" can have a negative connotation... http://mic.com/articles/127821/the-surprising-way-these-activists-are-using-veganism-to-fight-white-supremacy

"It's not merely that the most common rationale used..." pattrice jones, *The Oxen at the Intersection: A Collision*, Lantern Books, 2014, page 154. pattrice adds that disability rights activist Mary Fantaske goes even further, arguing that ableism and speciesism are the same thing. You can view Mary's presentation online at www.youtube.com/watch?v=6gGC2Z93xXk

**Research shows that ethical vegans...** Massimo Filippi, Gianna Riccitelli, Andrea Falini, Francesco Di Salle, Patrik Vuilleumier, Giancarlo Comi, Maria A. Rocca, "The Brain Functional Networks Associated to Human and Animal Suffering Differ among Omnivores, Vegetarians and Vegans," *PLOS One*, May 26, 2010.

**...increases our happiness and health...** www.ncbi.nlm.nih .gov/pmc/articles/PMC3156028/

**...makes us less inclined to be fearful of life's pains.** http://cercor.oxfordjournals.org/content/23/7/1552

**It also doubles your body's level of DHEA...** T.W. Pace, L.T. Negi, D.D. Adame, et al., "Effect of compassion meditation on neuroendocrine, innate immune and behavioral responses to psychosocial stress," *Psychoneuroendocrinology*, Volume 34, Number 1, 2009, pages 87–98.

**A study by Sara Konrath...** www.apa.org/news/press/rel eases/2011/09/volunteering-health.aspx

**...as was illustrated by a study that measured a phenomenon known as...** C. Daryl Cameron and B. Keith Payne, "Escaping affect: How motivated emotion regulation creates insensitivity to mass suffering," *Journal of Personality and Social Psychology*, Volume 100, Number 1, January 2011.

**This intrigued researchers at Stanford University...** Karina Schumann, Jamil Zaki, and Carol S. Dweck, "Addressing the empathy deficit: Beliefs about the malleability of empathy predict effortful responses when empathy is challenging," *Journal of Personality and Social Psychology*, Volume 107, Number 3, September 2014, pages 475–93.

**Researchers Barbara Fredrickson and Steve Cole...** www.pnas.org/content/110/33/13684.full

**In yet another study...** Jared Piazza, Matthew B. Ruby, Steve Loughnan, Mischel Luong, Juliana Kulik, Hanne M. Watkins, Mirra Seigerman, "Rationalizing meat consumption: The 4Ns,"

*Appetite*, Volume 91, August 1, 2015.

**...how sexist people also have racist tendencies...** Maite Garaigordobil y Jone Aliri, "Sexismo hostil y benevolente: relaciones con el autoconcepto, el racismo y la sensibilidad intercultural," *Revista de Psicodidáctica*, Volume 16, Number 2, 2011, pages 331–50.

**I am reminded of a video...** www.youtube.com/watch?v=2K lmvmuxzYE

## Chapter 6: Q & A

**...about 80 percent of all antibiotics are currently used on farmed animals...** www.foodandwaterwatch.org/reports/antibio tic-resistance-101-how-antibiotic-misuse-on-factory-farms-can-make-you-sick/

**Recent research has indicated that plants respond...** Michael Pollan, "The Intelligent Plant," *The New Yorker*, December 23, 2013.

**...70 percent of crops go to feed farmed animals...** www.worldwatch.org/node/549

**With some 70 billion land animals butchered for human consumption worldwide every year...** www.ciwf.org.uk/me dia/3640540/ciwf_strategic_plan_20132017.pdf

# Select Index

# About the Author

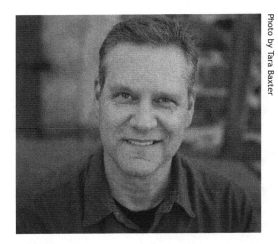

Photo by Tara Baxter

Mark Hawthorne is an activist and the author of two other books on animal rights: *Bleating Hearts: The Hidden World of Animal Suffering* and *Striking at the Roots: A Practical Guide to Animal Activism* (both from Changemakers Books). He stopped eating meat after an encounter with one of India's many cows in 1992 and became an ethical vegan a decade later. In addition to his work in such publications as *VegNews*, *The Vegan*, and *Laika*, his writing has been featured in *Vegan's Daily Companion* (Quarry Books), *SATYA: The Long View* (Lantern Books), *Uncaged: Top Activists Share Their Wisdom on Effective Farm Animal Advocacy* (Ben Davidow), and *Turning Points in Compassion* (SpiritWings Humane Education Inc.), as well as in the anthologies *Stories to Live By: Wisdom to Help You Make the Most of Every Day* and *The Best Travel Writing 2005: True Stories from Around the World* (both from Travelers' Tales). Mark and his wife lauren live in California. You'll find him tweeting @markhawthorne.

MarkHawthorne.com
Facebook.com/MarkHawthorneAuthor

# Other Changemakers Books by Mark Hawthorne

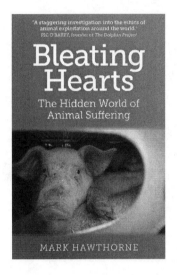

*Bleating Hearts: The Hidden World of Animal Suffering*

Comprehensive and hard-hitting, *Bleating Hearts* examines the world's vast exploitation of animals, from the food, fashion, and research industries to the use of other species for sport, war, entertainment, religion, labor, and pleasure.

In the face of information that might render us speechless, Mark Hawthorne is thorough and articulate. *Bleating Hearts* empowers us with ways to challenge what has been both normal and hidden, making this book a remarkable achievement of vision and voice.
**Carol J. Adams**, author of *The Sexual Politics of Meat*

If there is a place in your heart for animals, this is an important book for you to read. But it is also more than that. If you want to lift the veil of denial, so that you can make your life an effective statement of compassion, you'll find this book to be nothing less than extraordinary.
**John Robbins**, author of *The Food Revolution* and *Diet For A New America* and co-founder of the Food Revolution Network

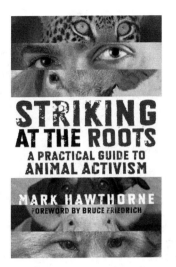

*Striking at the Roots: A Practical Guide to Animal Activism*

*Striking at the Roots: A Practical Guide to Animal Activism* brings together the most effective tactics for speaking out for animals and gives voice to activists from around the globe, who explain why their chosen models of activism have been successful—and how others can get involved.

If you are serious about helping animals, then you should seriously read this book.
**Captain Paul Watson**, founder of Sea Shepherd Conservation Society

This book motivates and informs, puts the passion into compassion and will save lives.
**Juliet Gellatley**, founder of Viva!